NURSE

COLORING BOOK

By Noah's Art

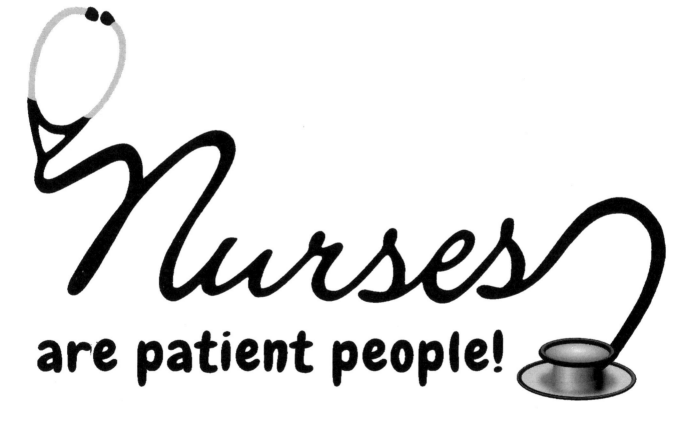

Nurses are patient people!

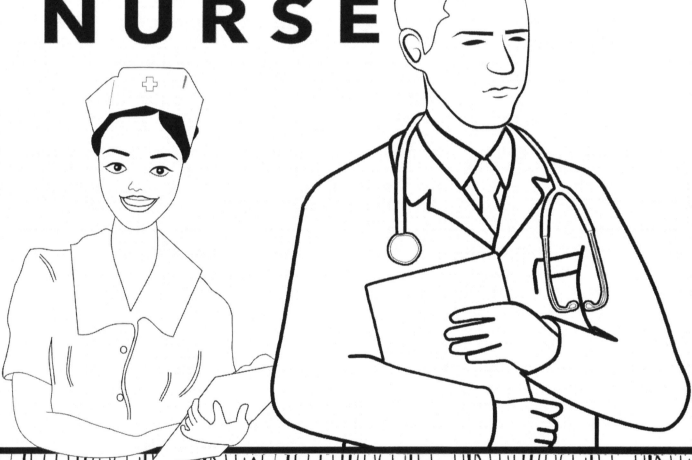

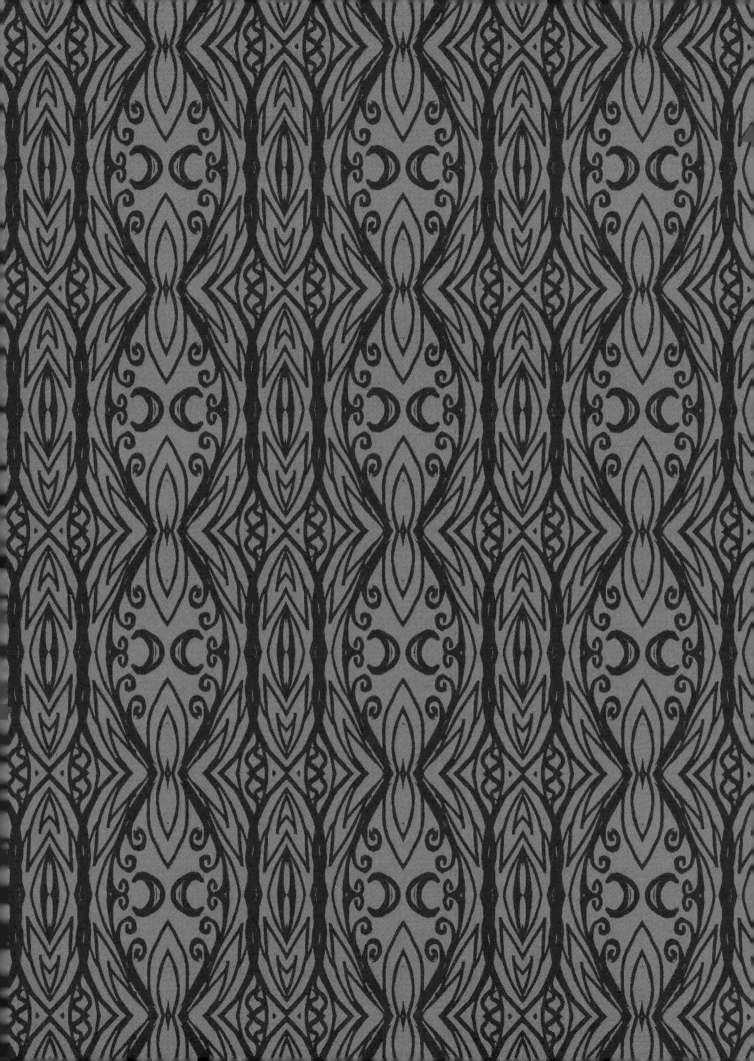

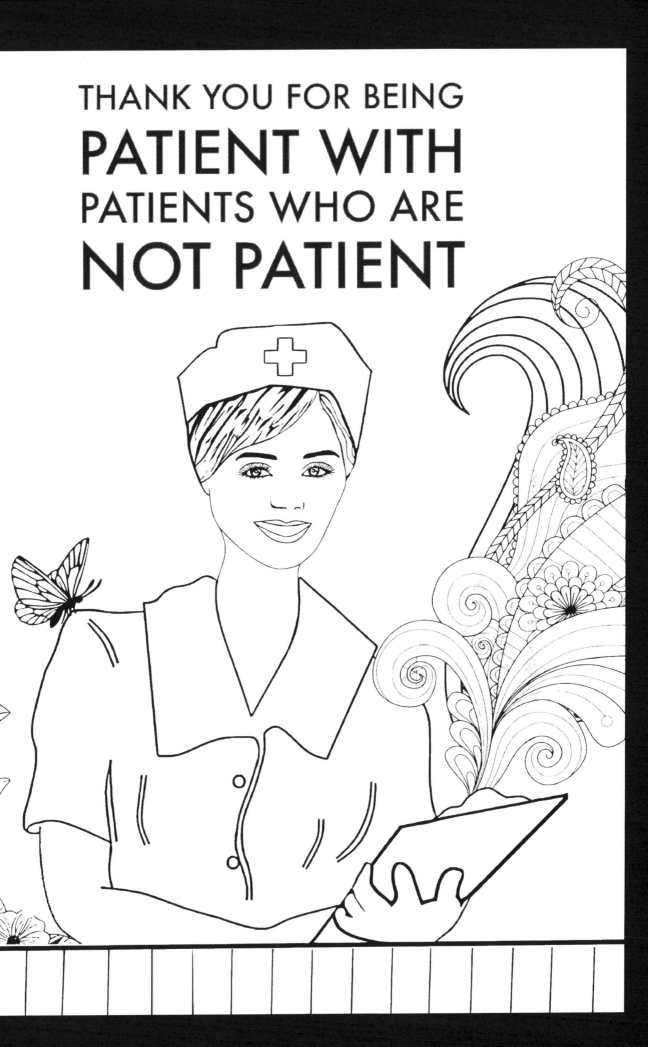

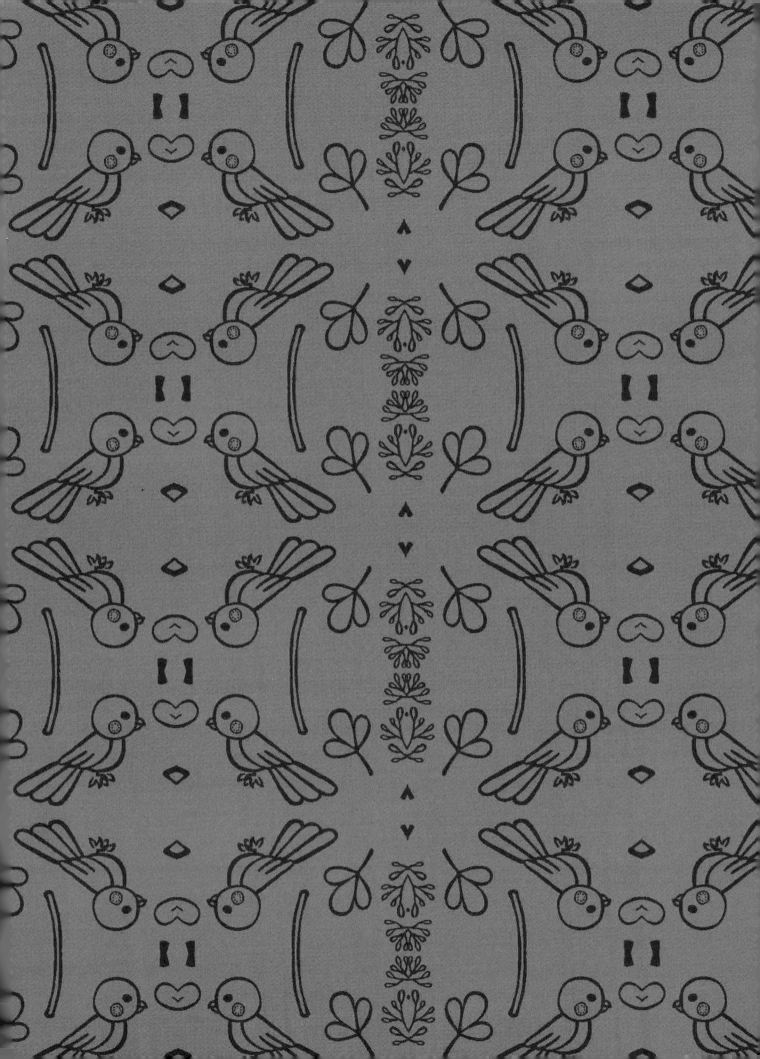

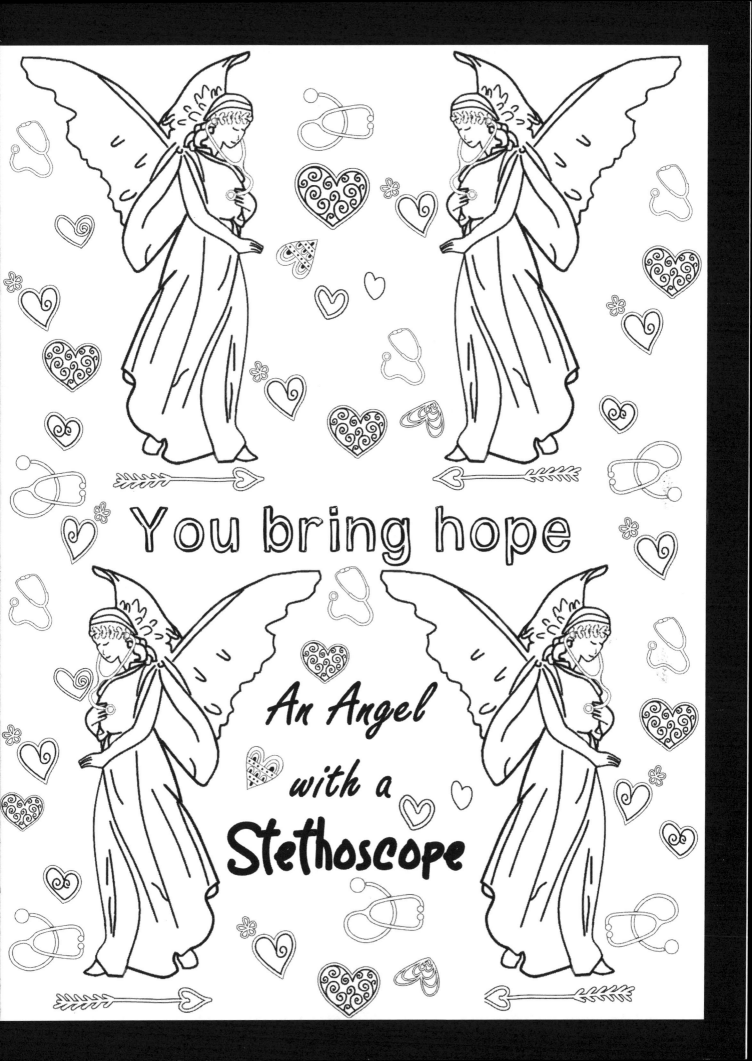

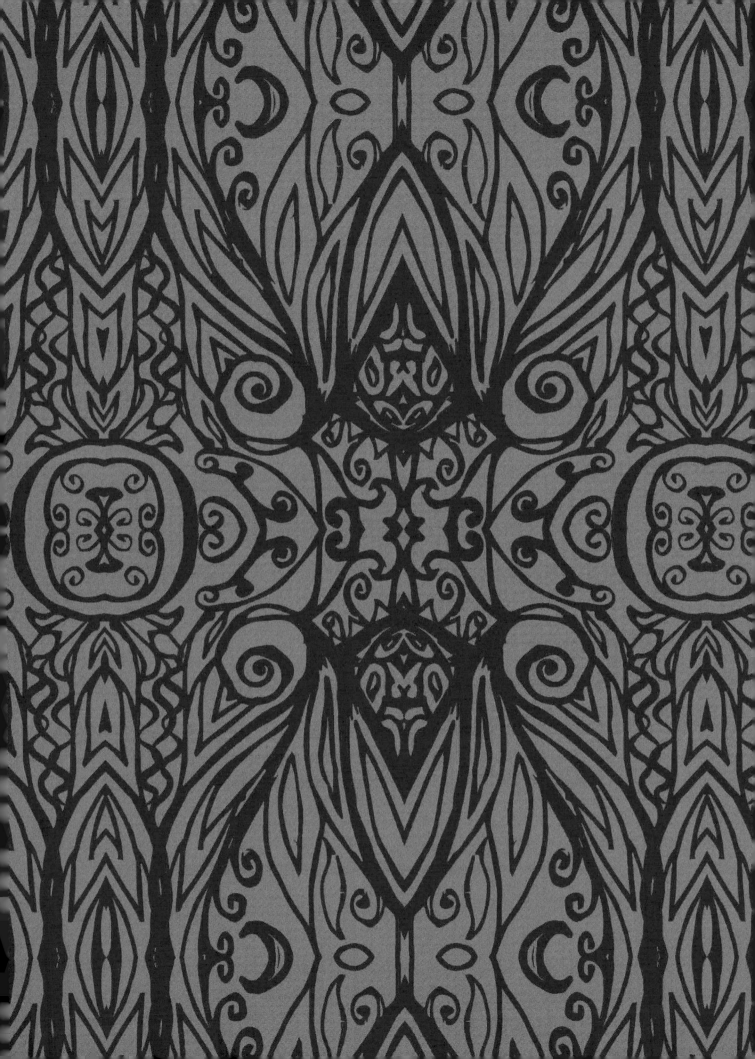

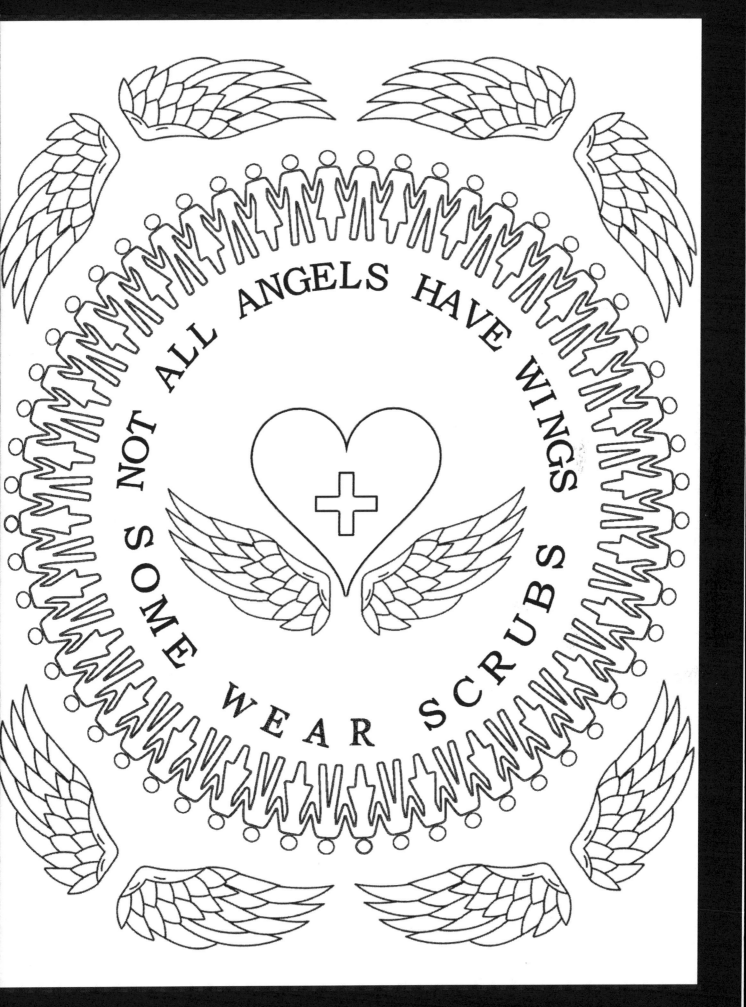

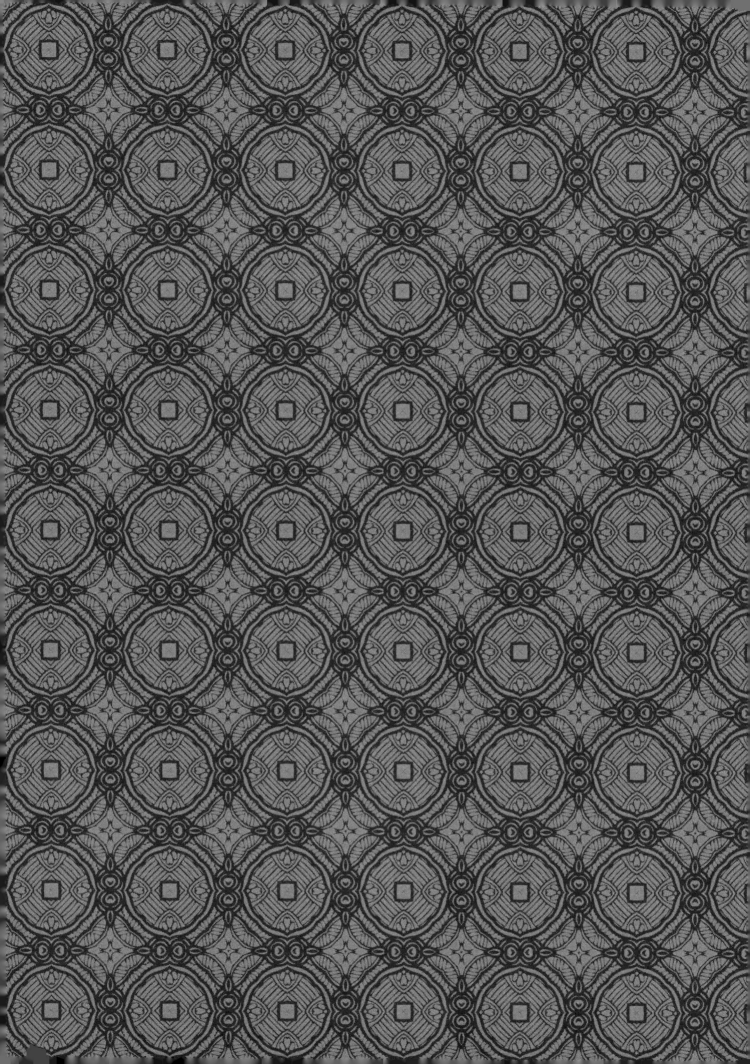

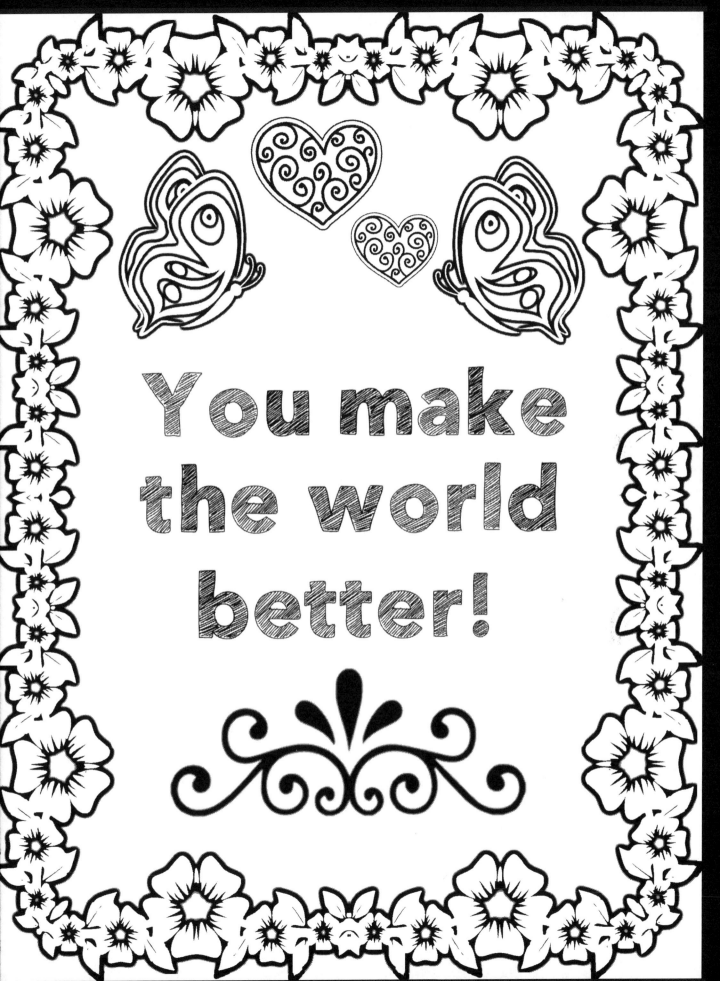

You make the world better!

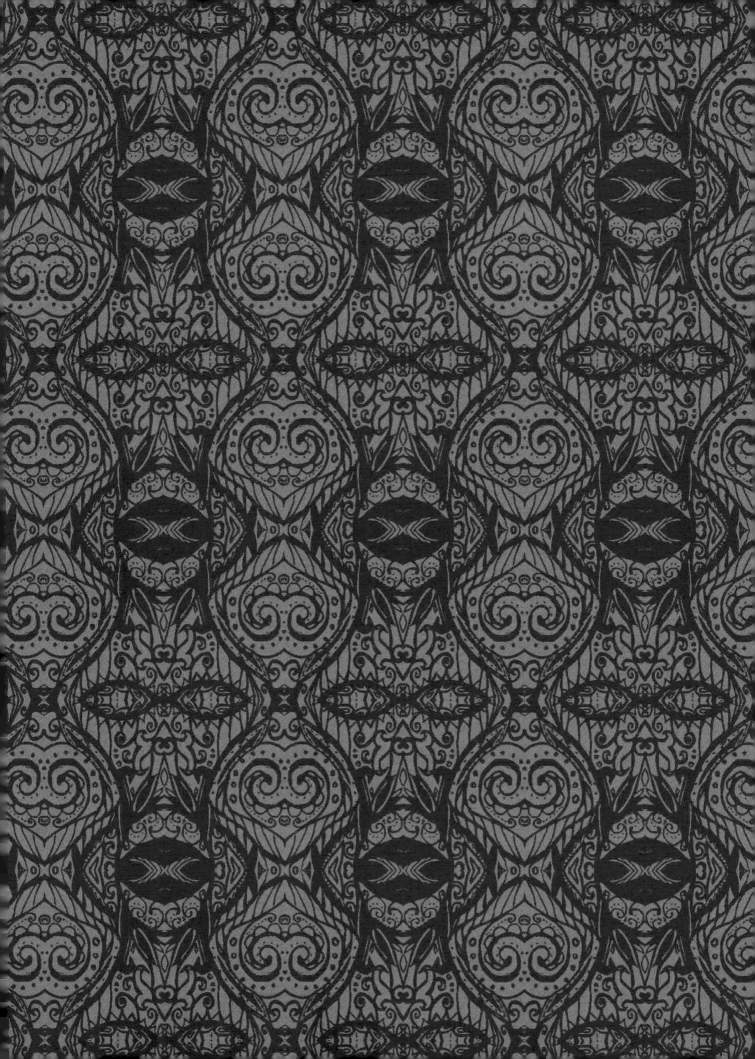

Nursing is
a work
of Heart

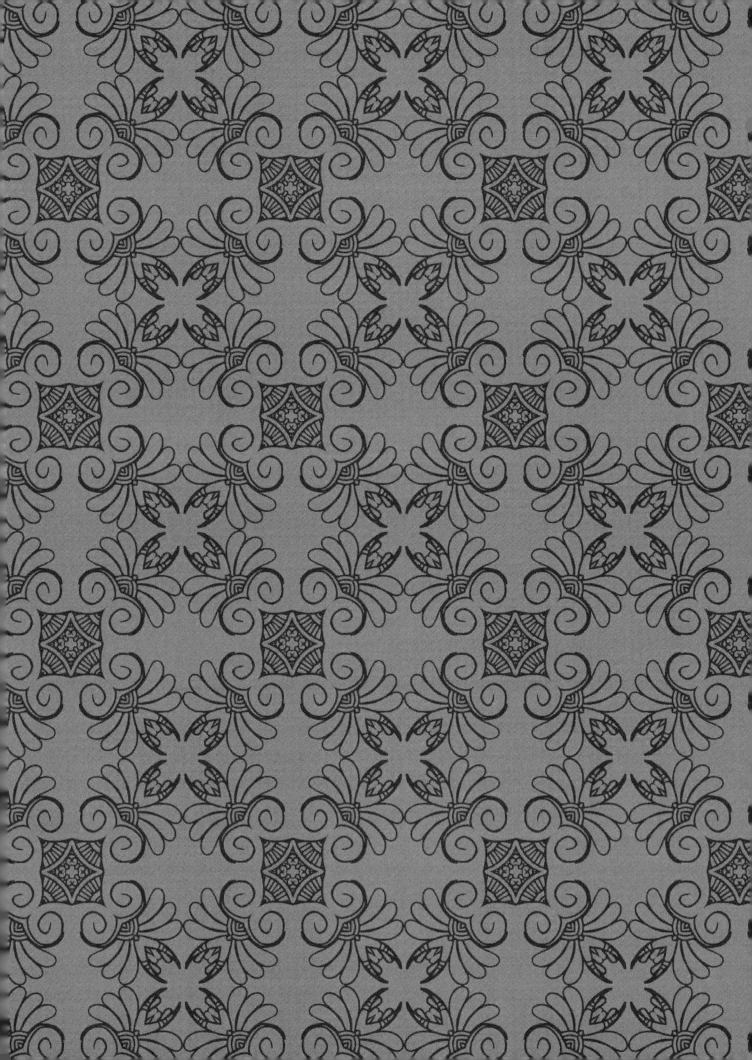

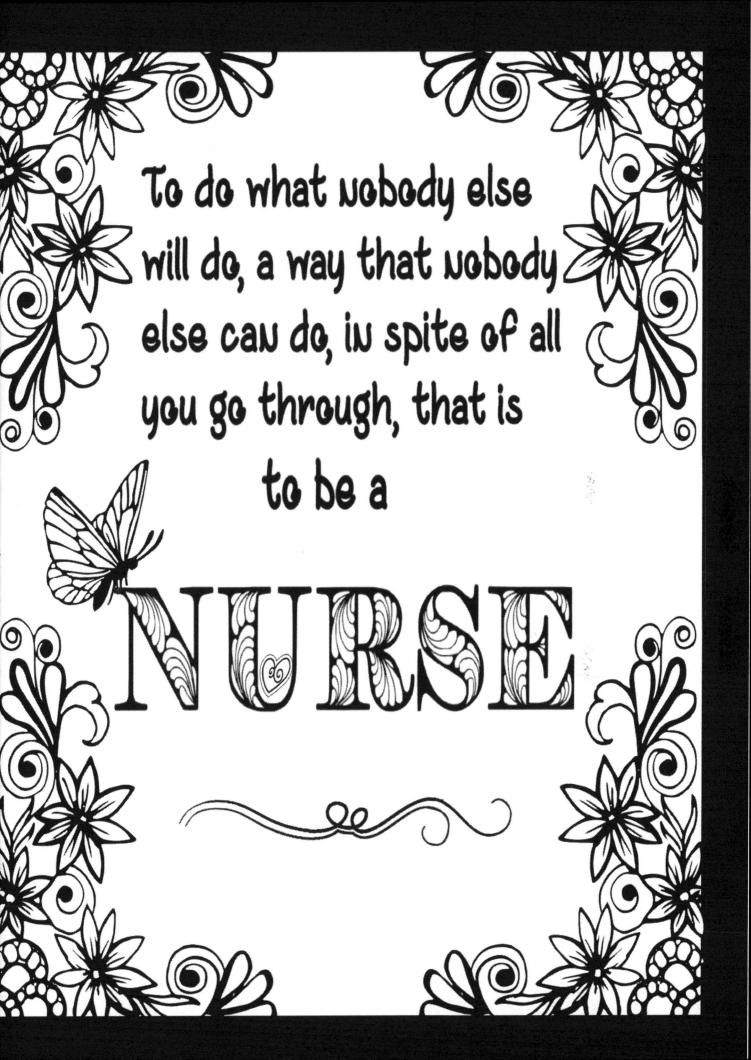

To do what nobody else will do, a way that nobody else can do, in spite of all you go through, that is to be a

NURSE

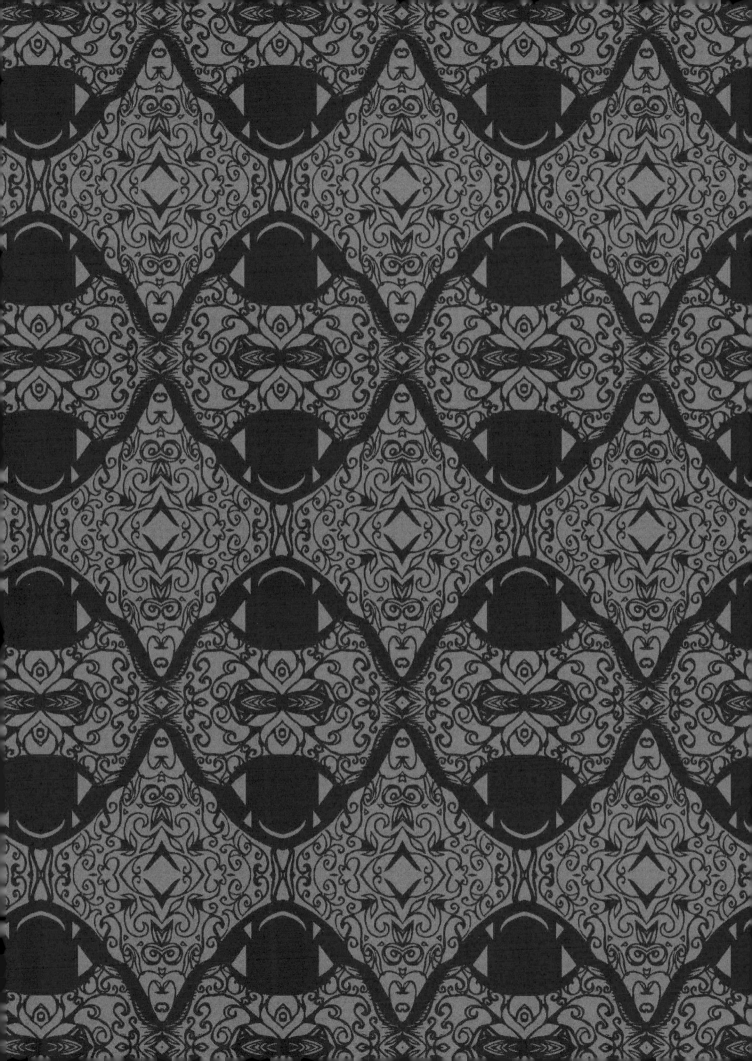

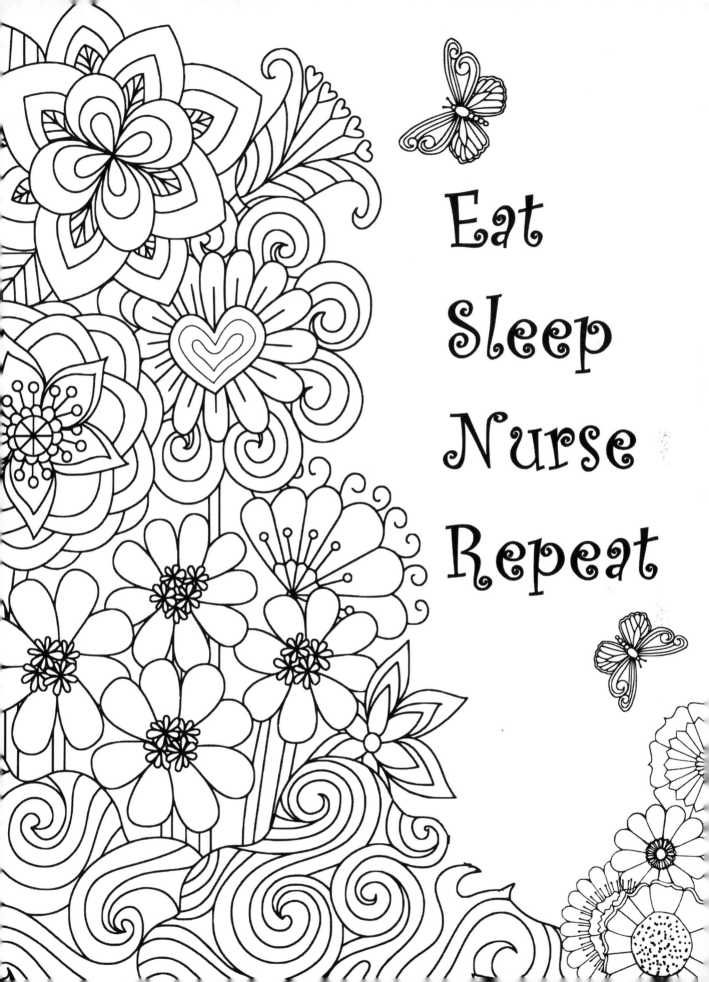

Eat
Sleep
Nurse
Repeat

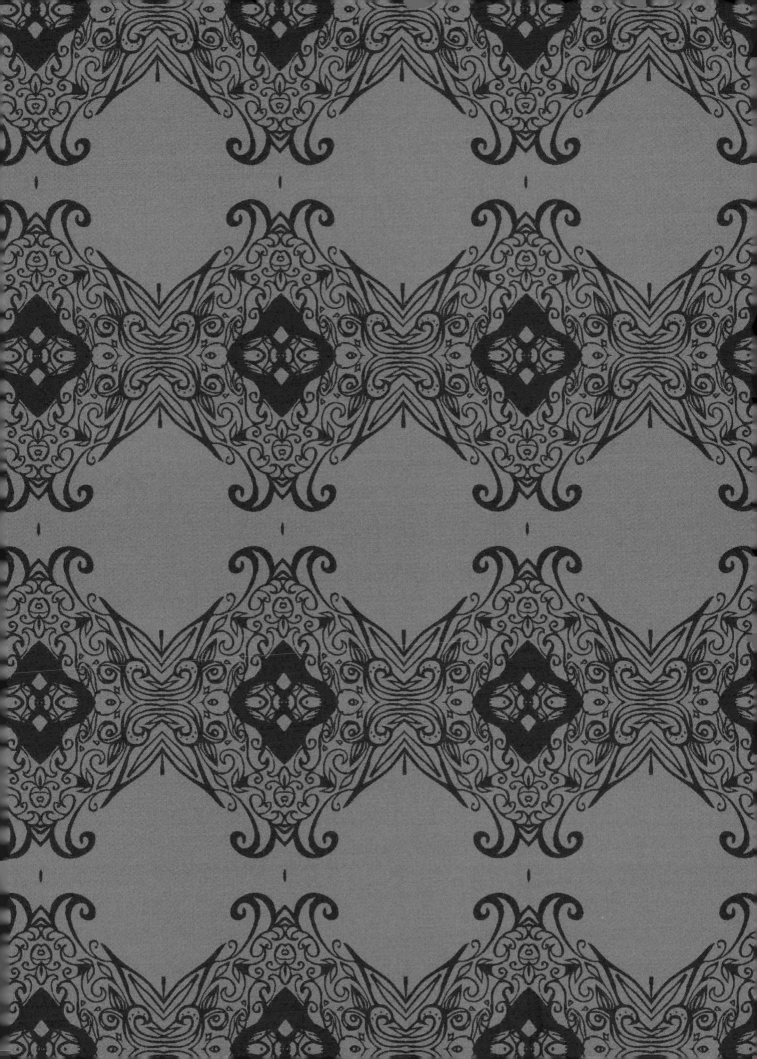

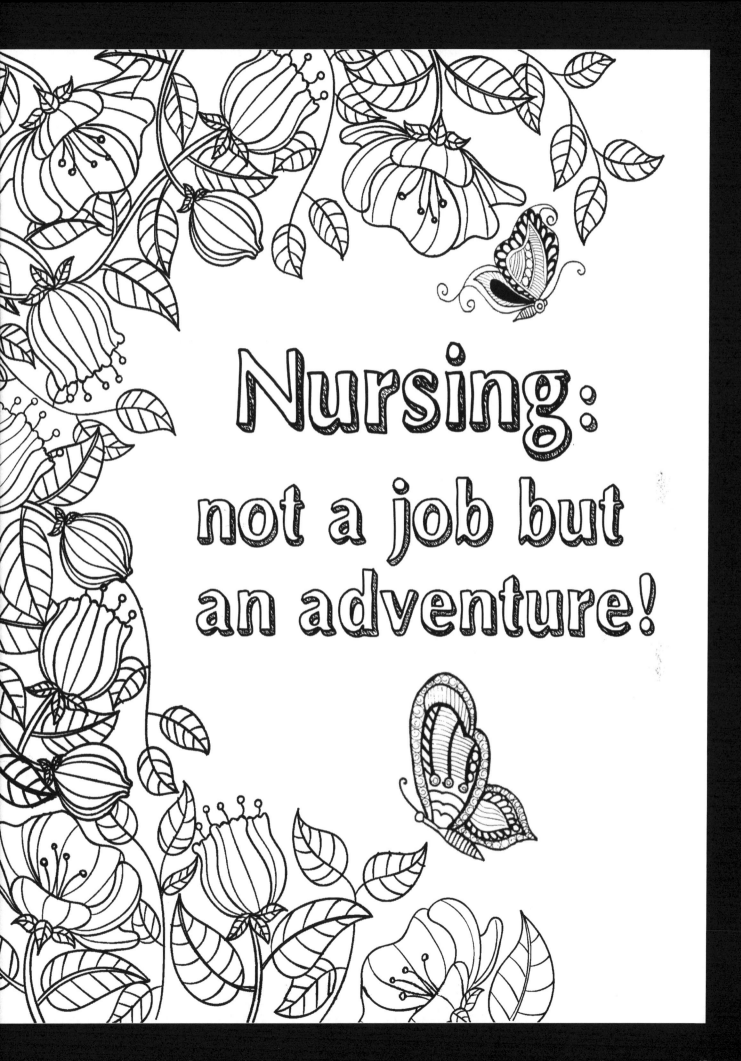

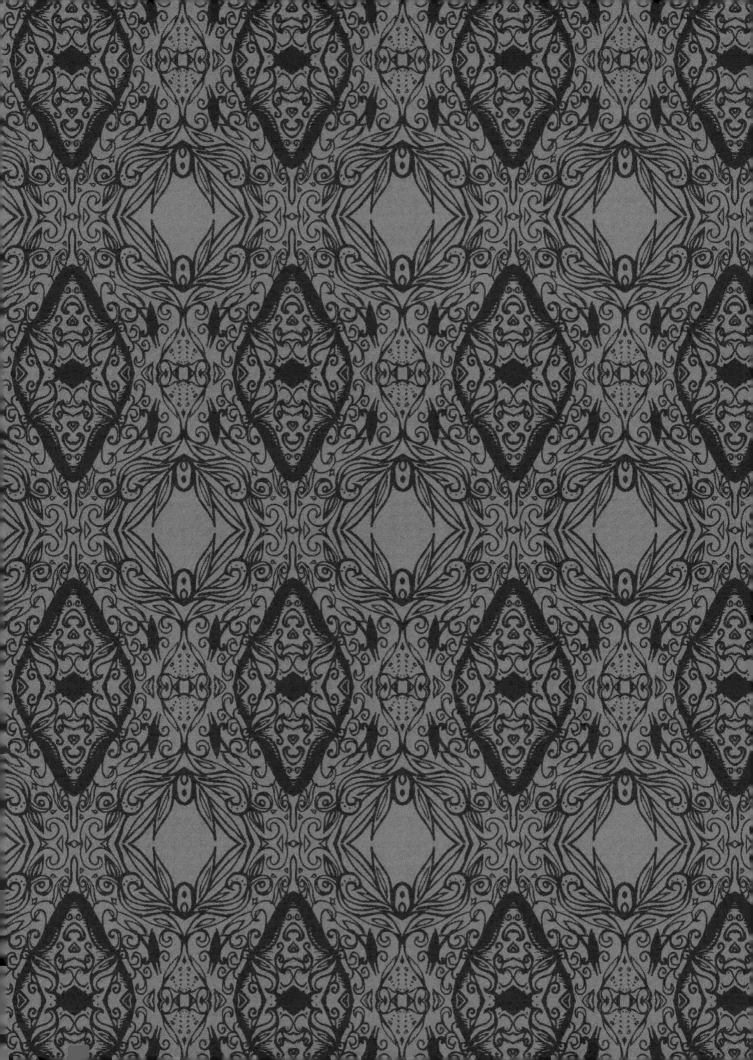

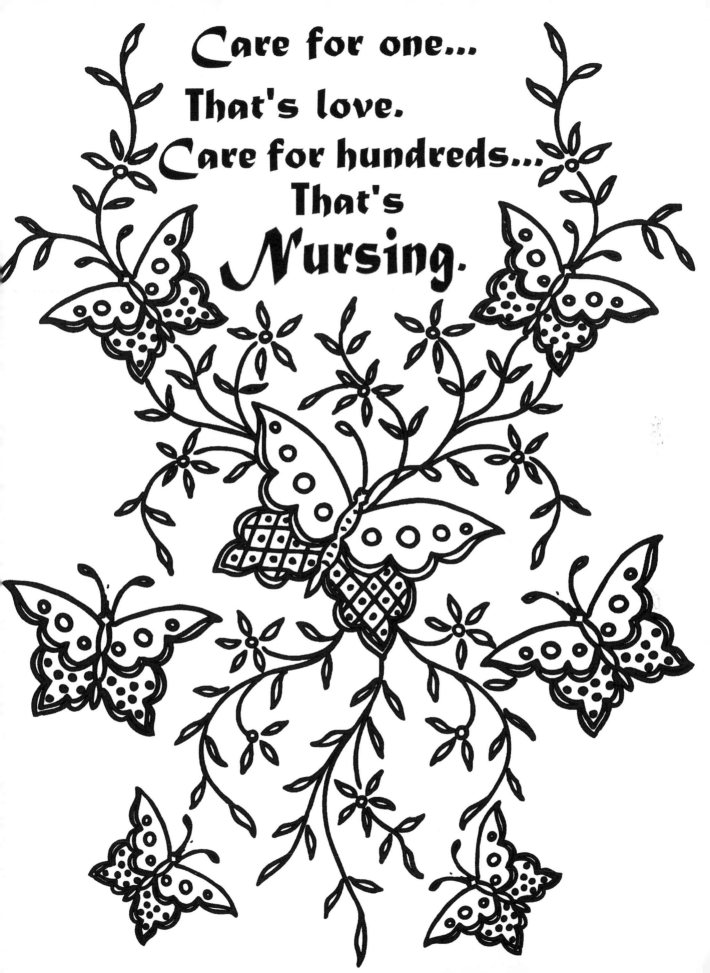

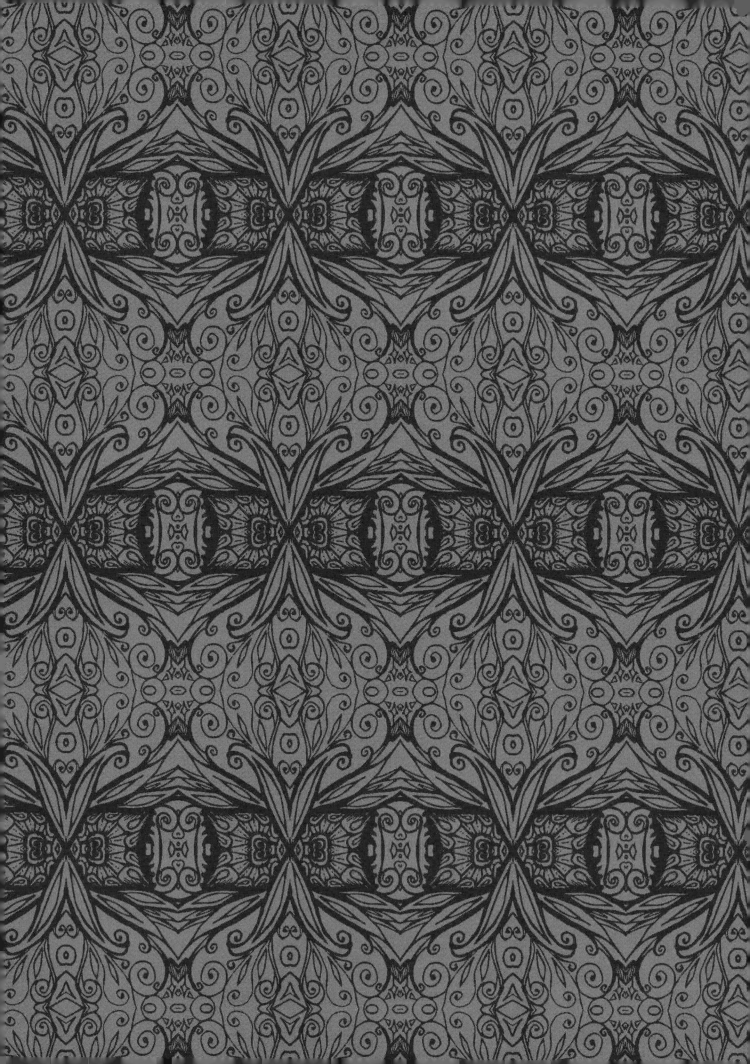

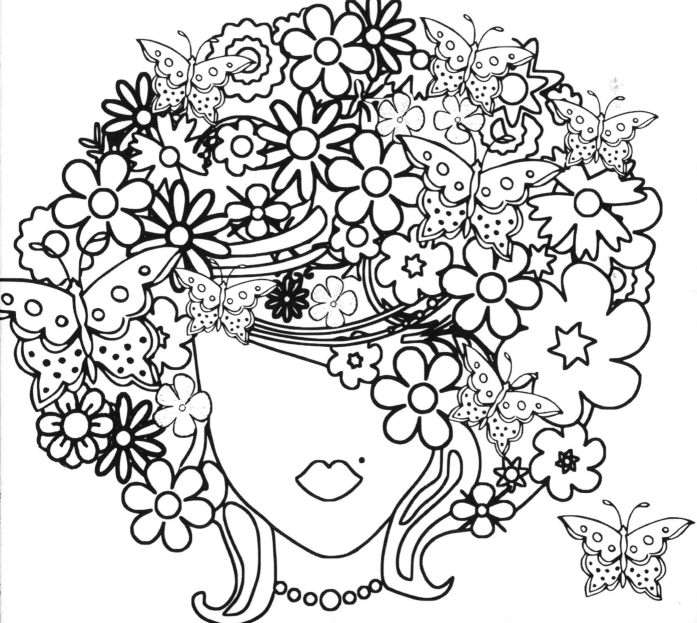

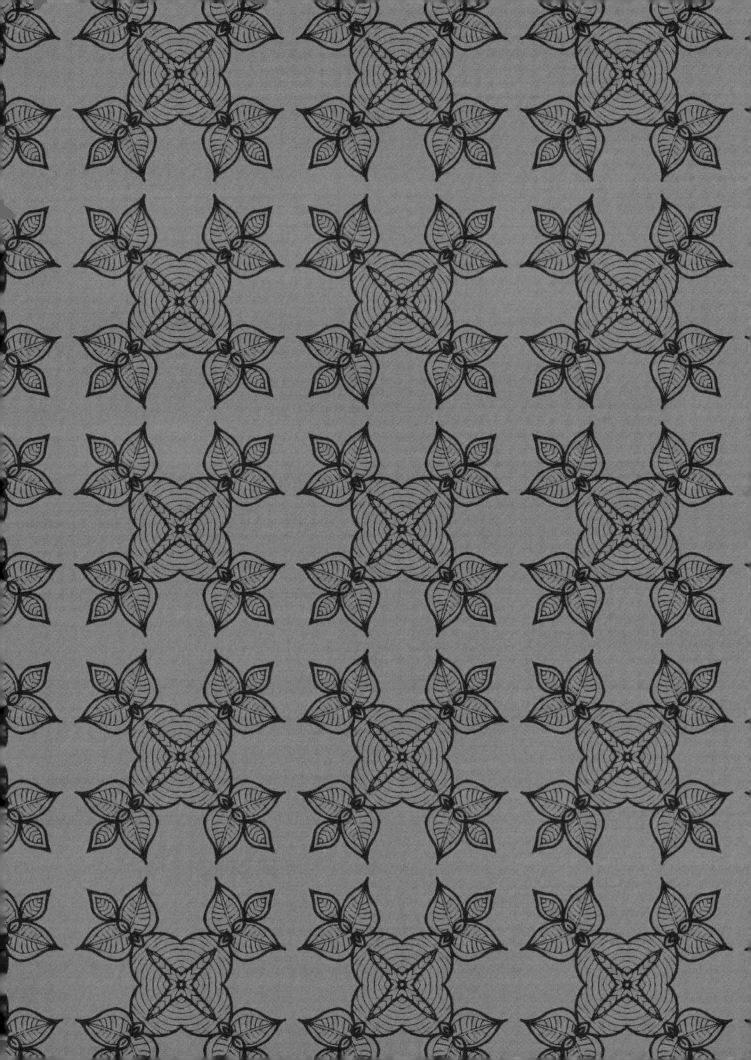

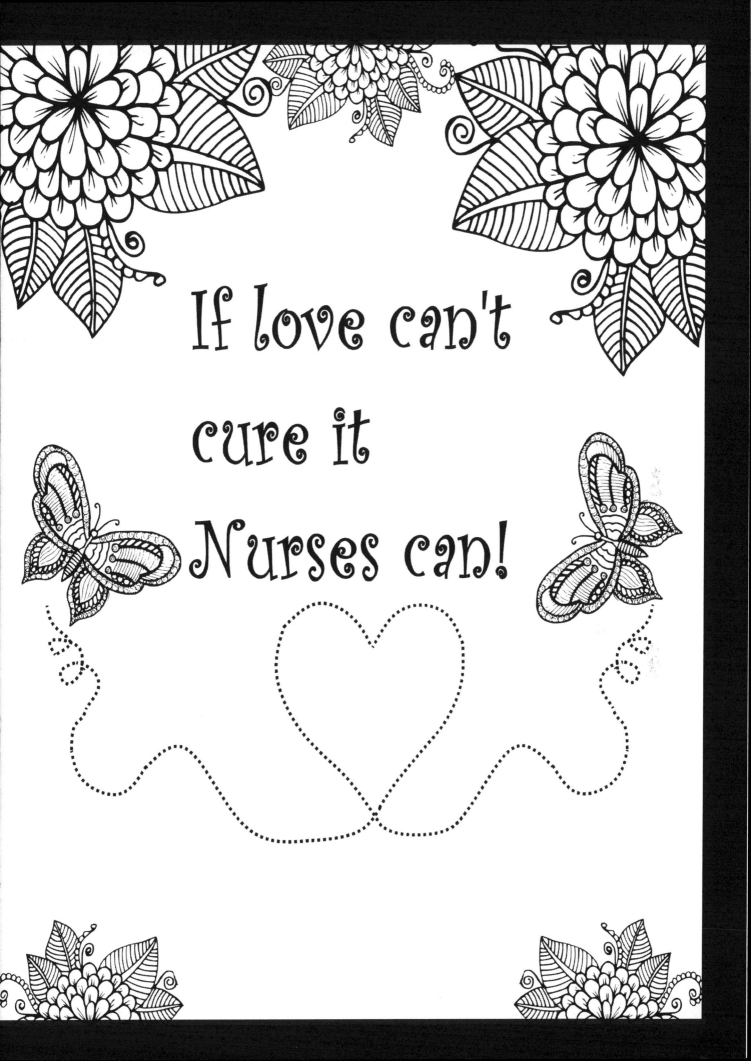

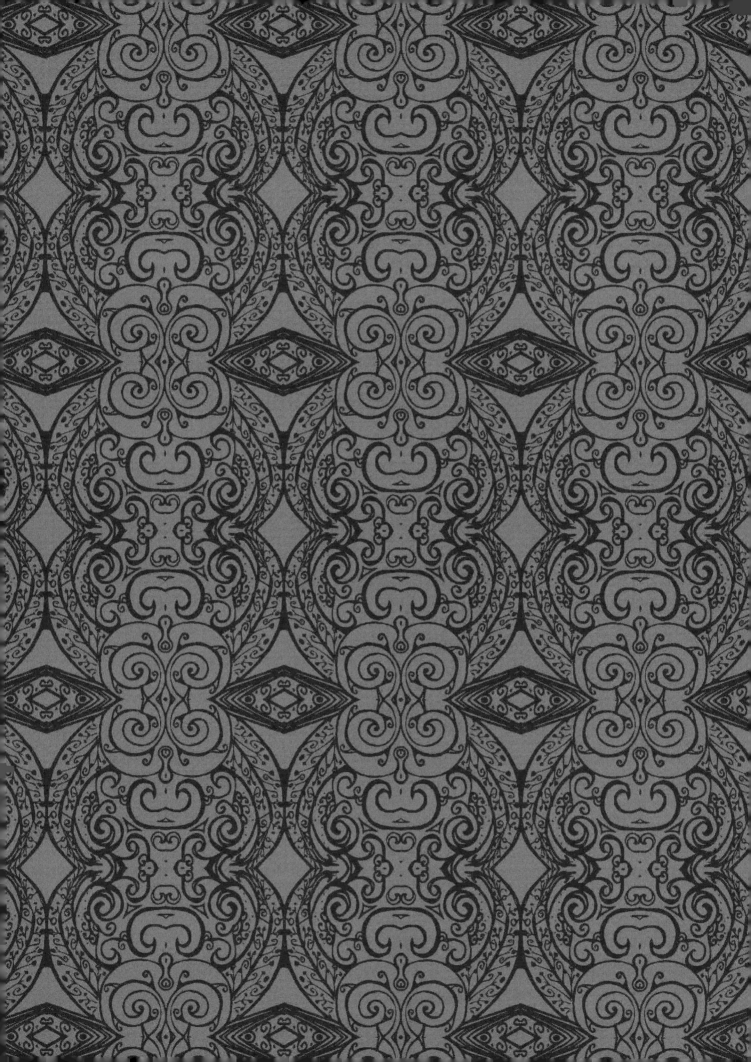

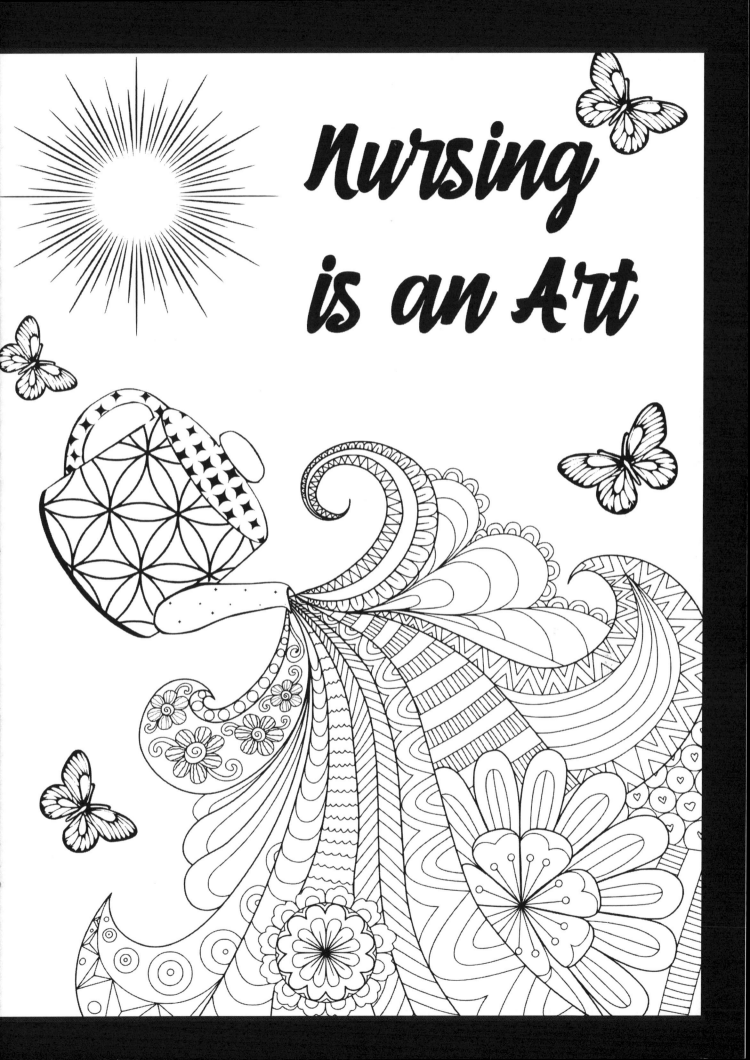

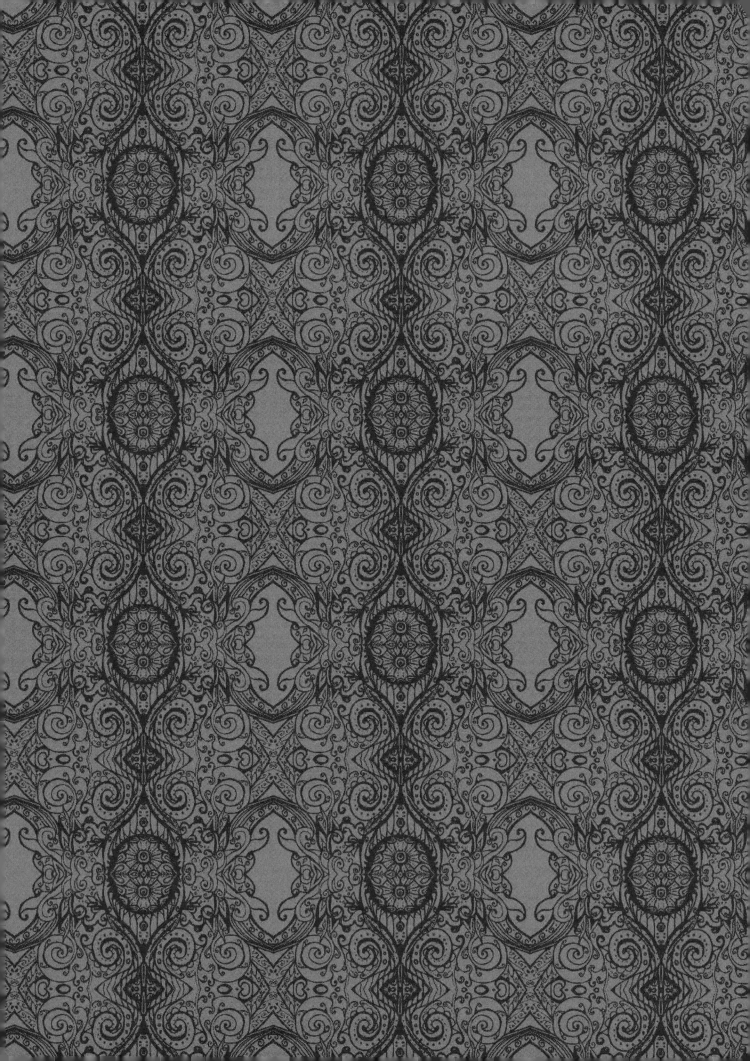

Nurses are the hospitality of the hospital.

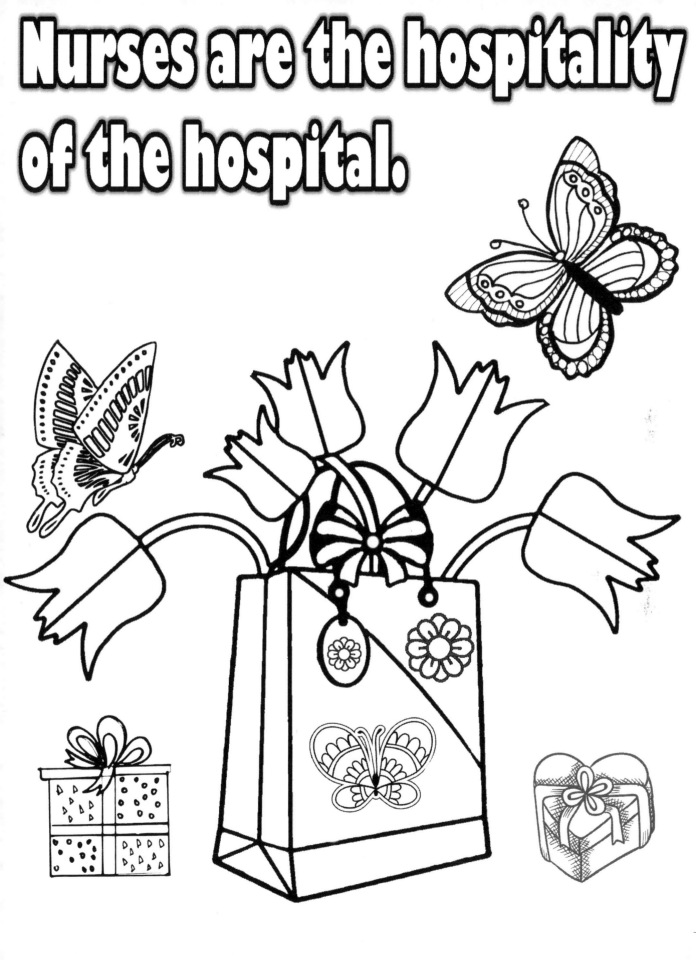

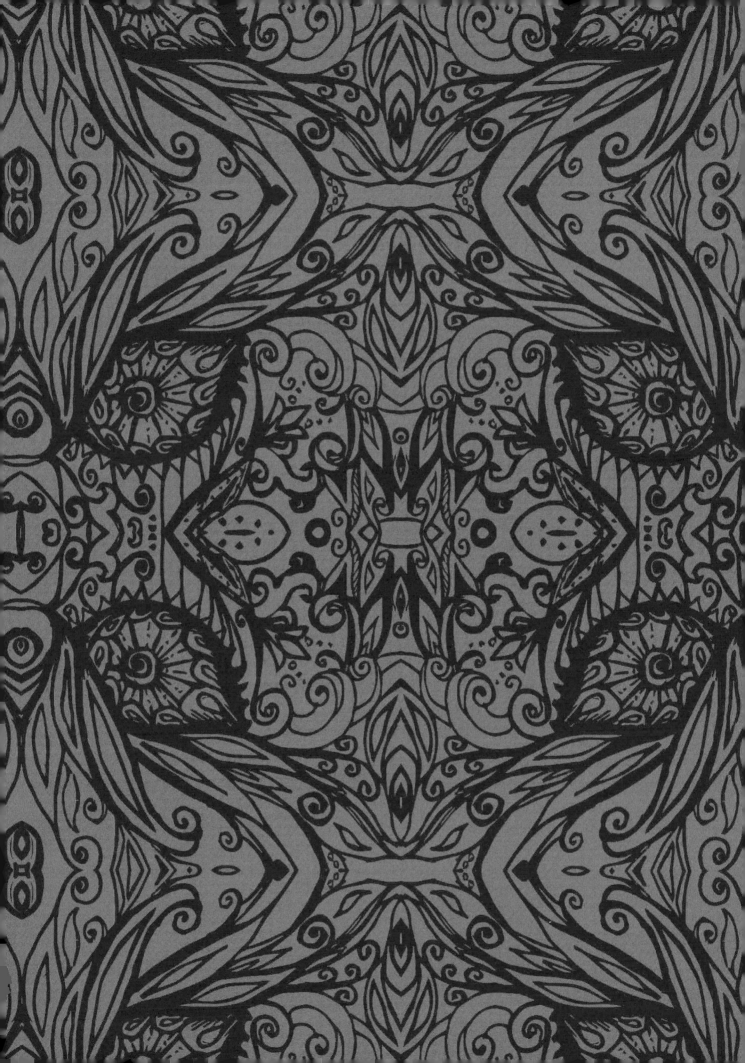

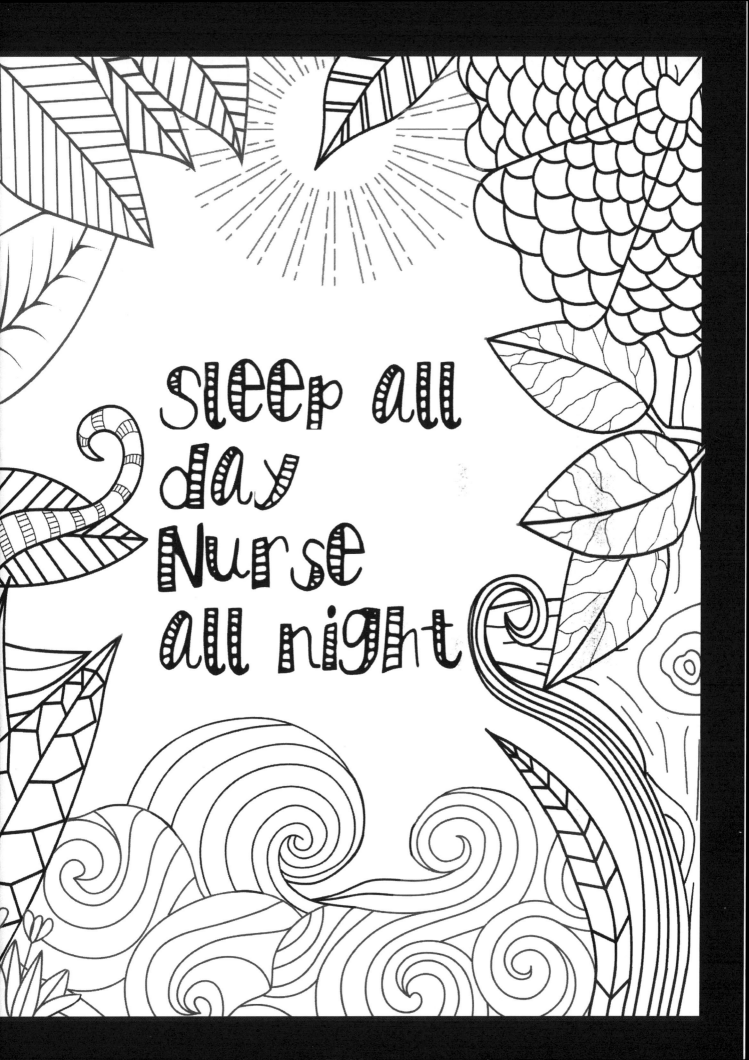

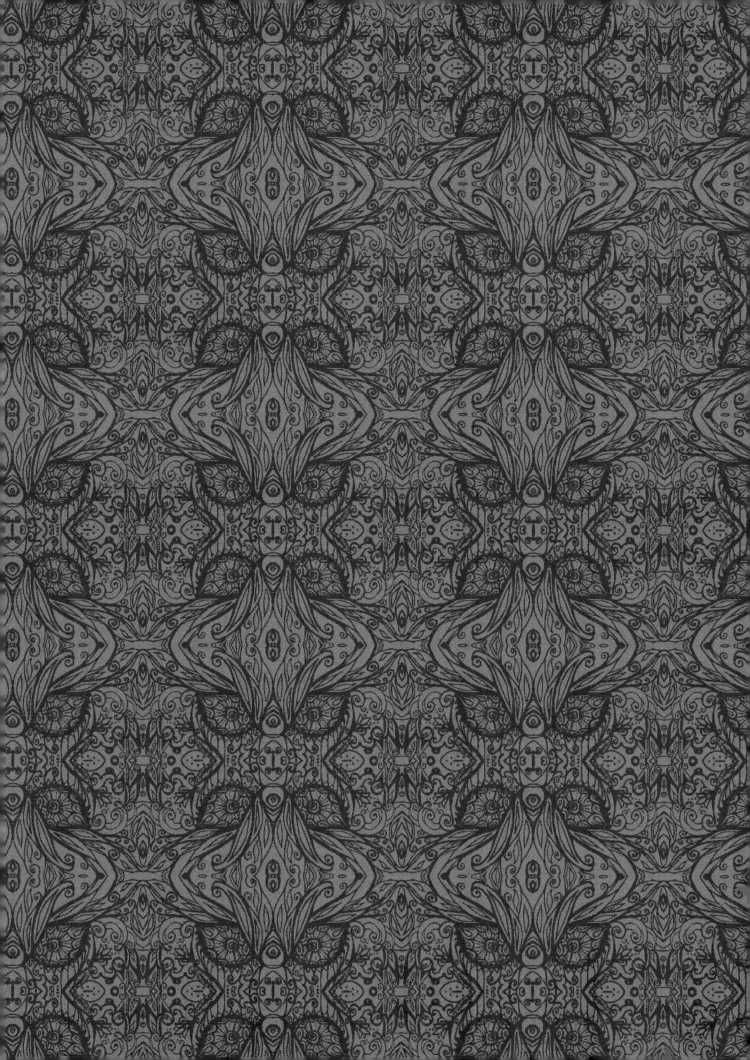

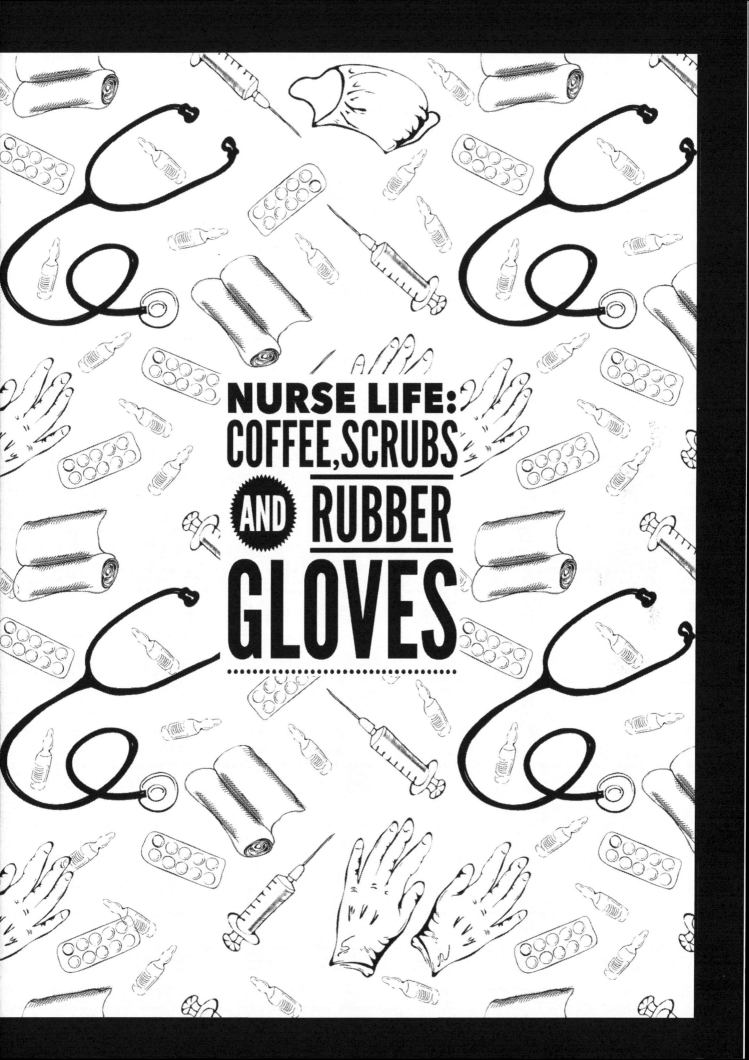

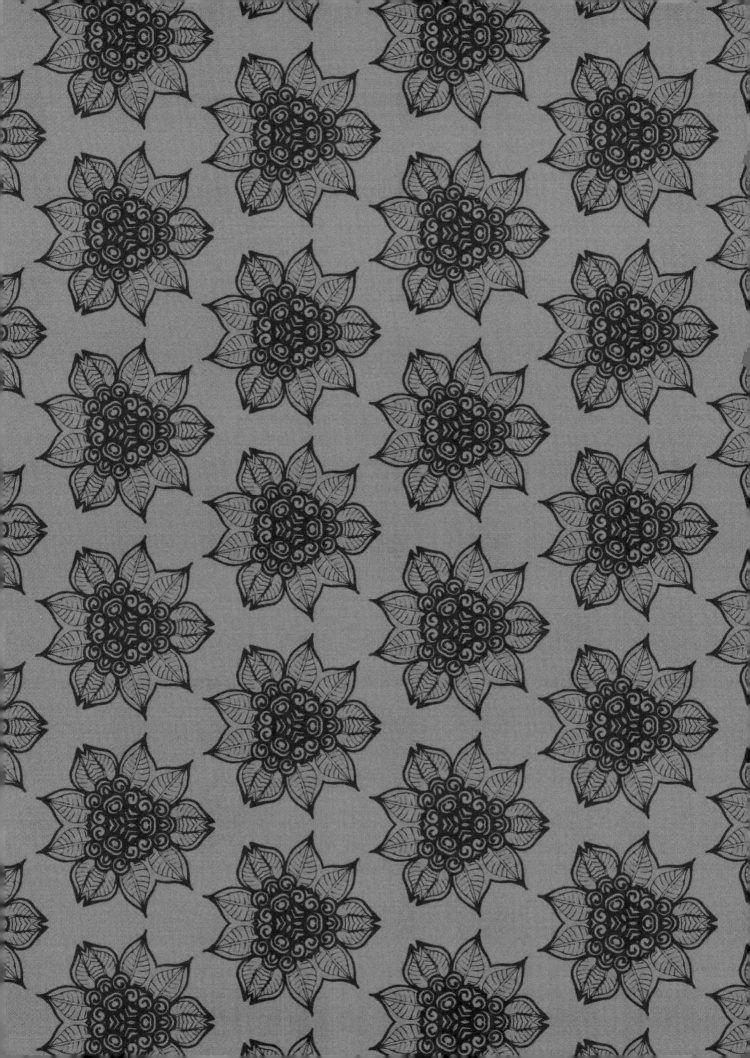

NURSE: THE PERSON who can drink a pot of coffee, go home and go to bed.

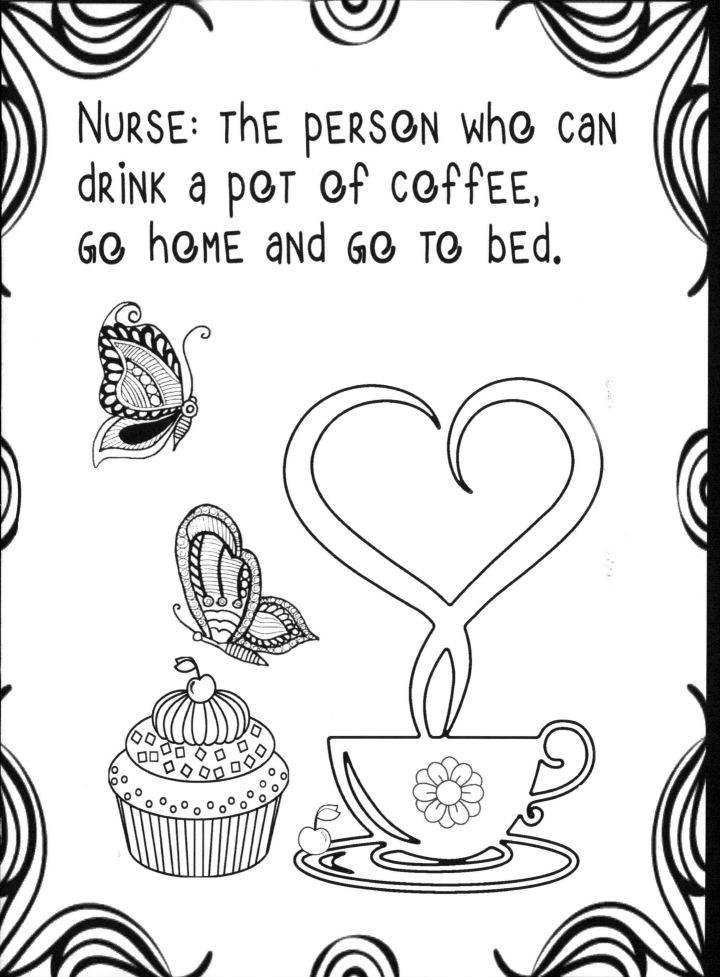

NURSES ARE COMPASSIONATE AND PATIENT PEOPLE

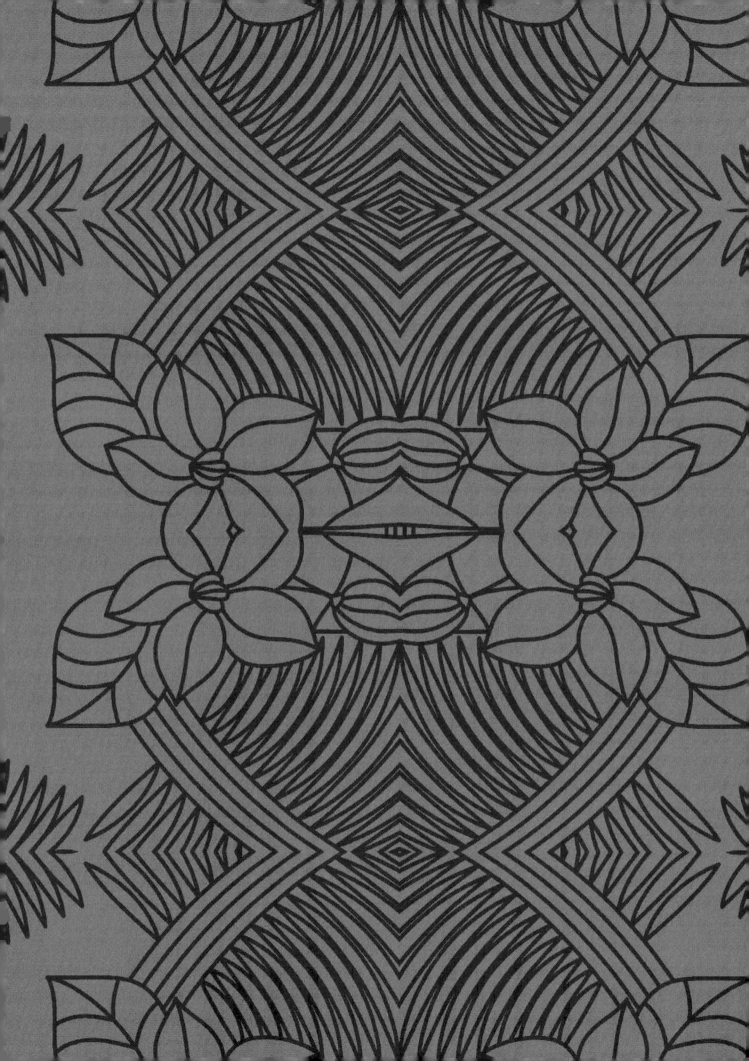

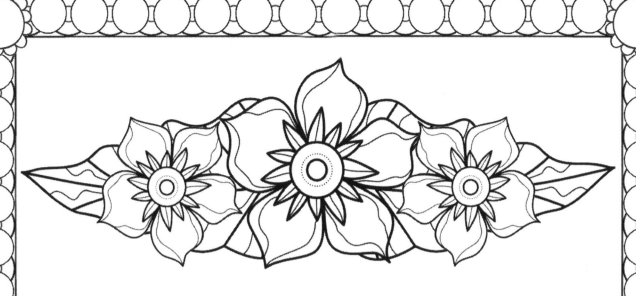

Nursing is the Gentle Art Of caring For others

Nursing: changing lives one smile at a time.

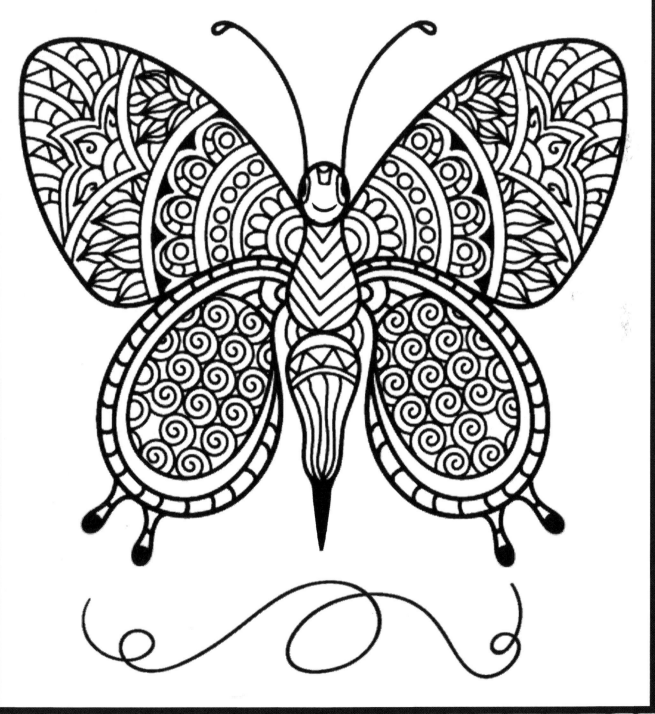

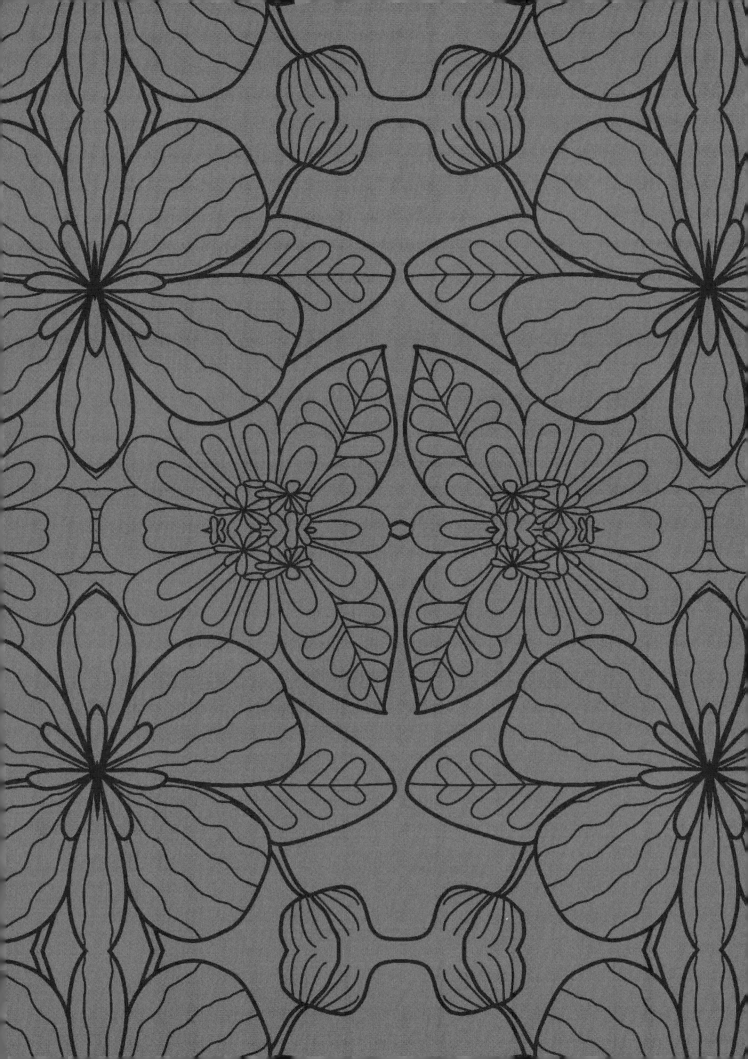

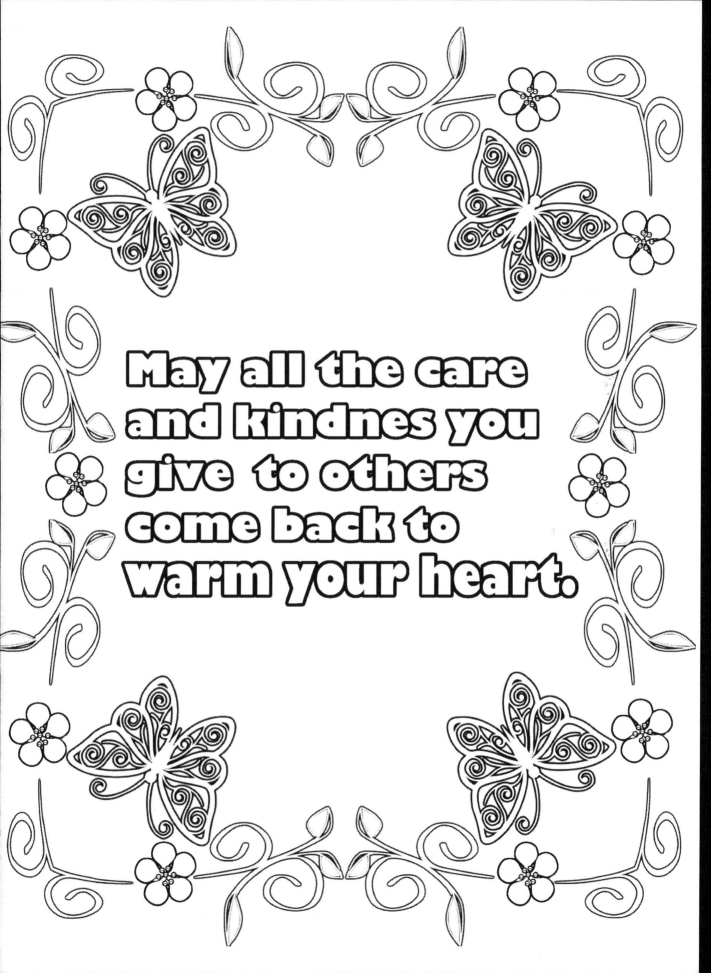

May all the care
and kindnes you
give to others
come back to
warm your heart.

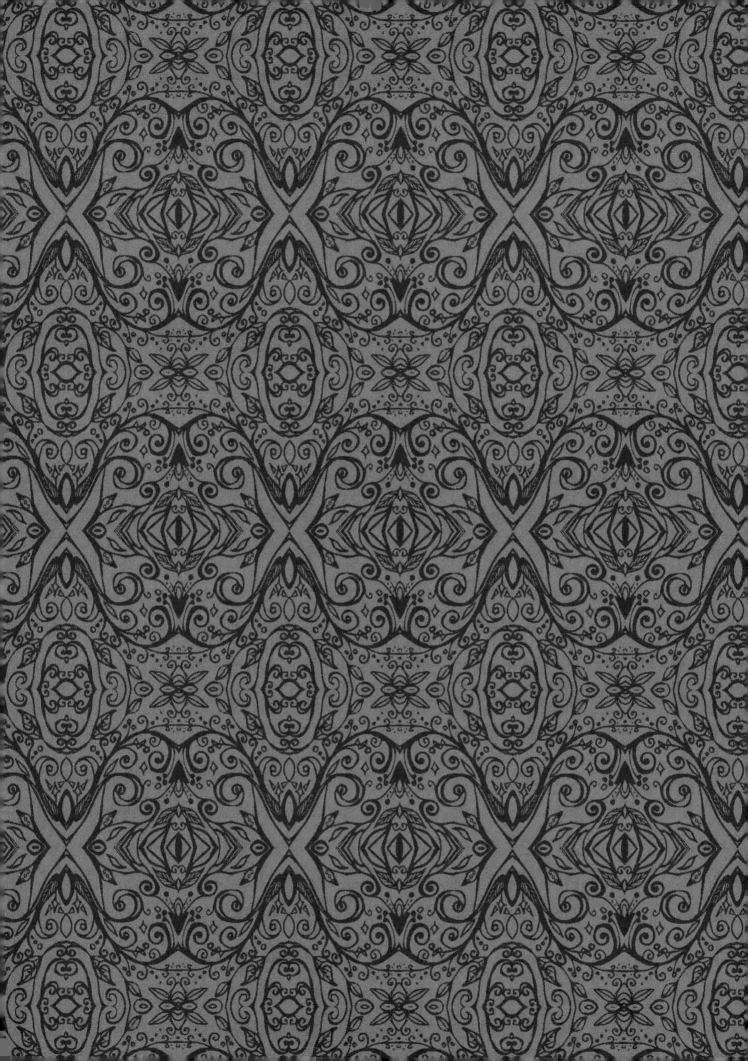

NURSES ARE ALL HEART

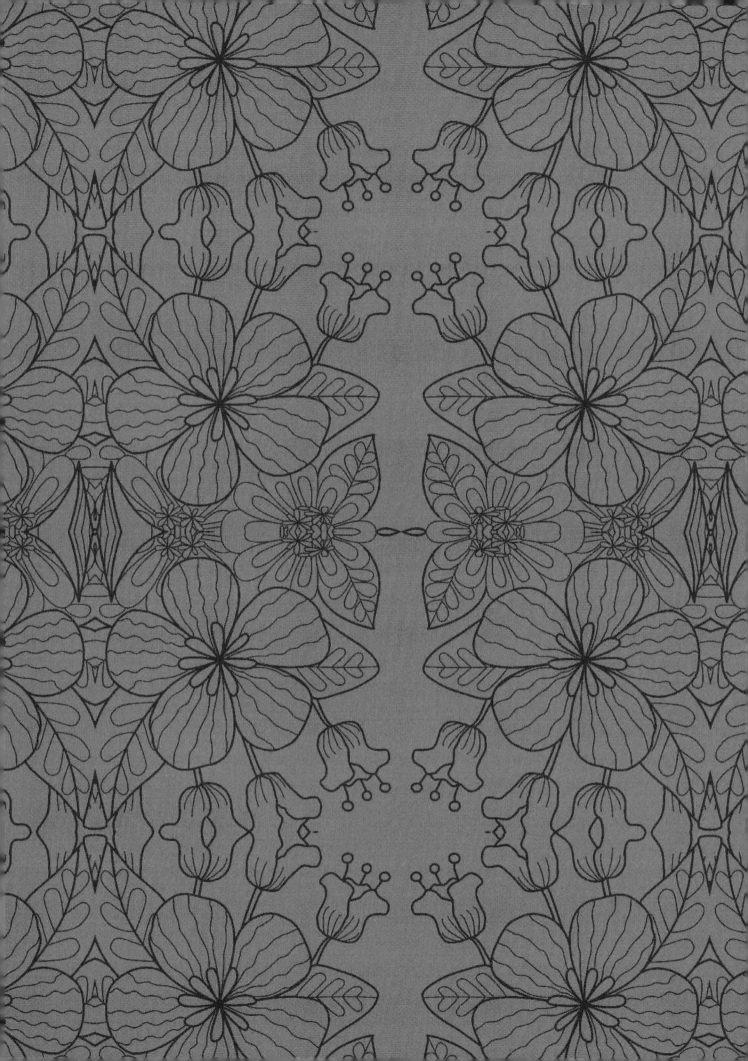

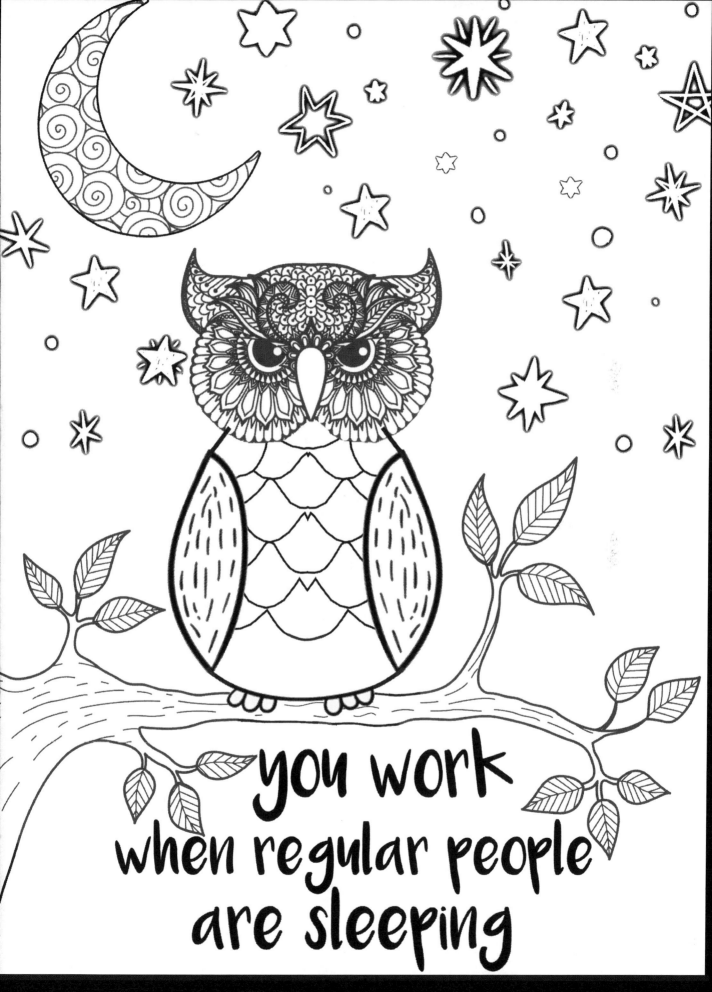

you work when regular people are sleeping

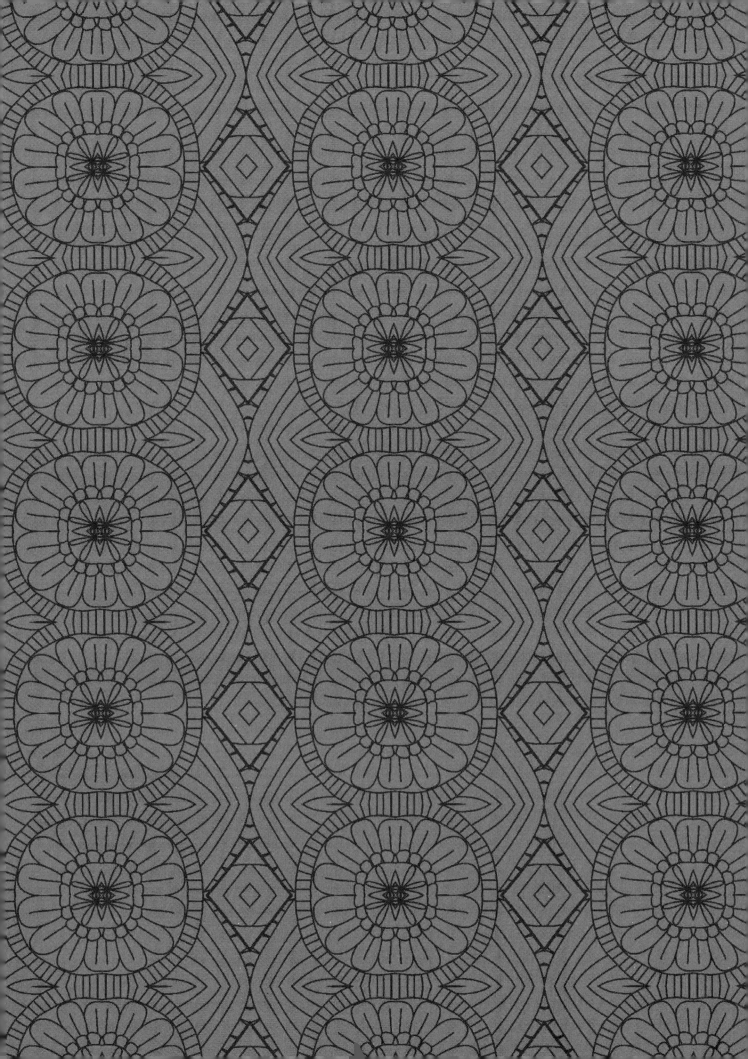

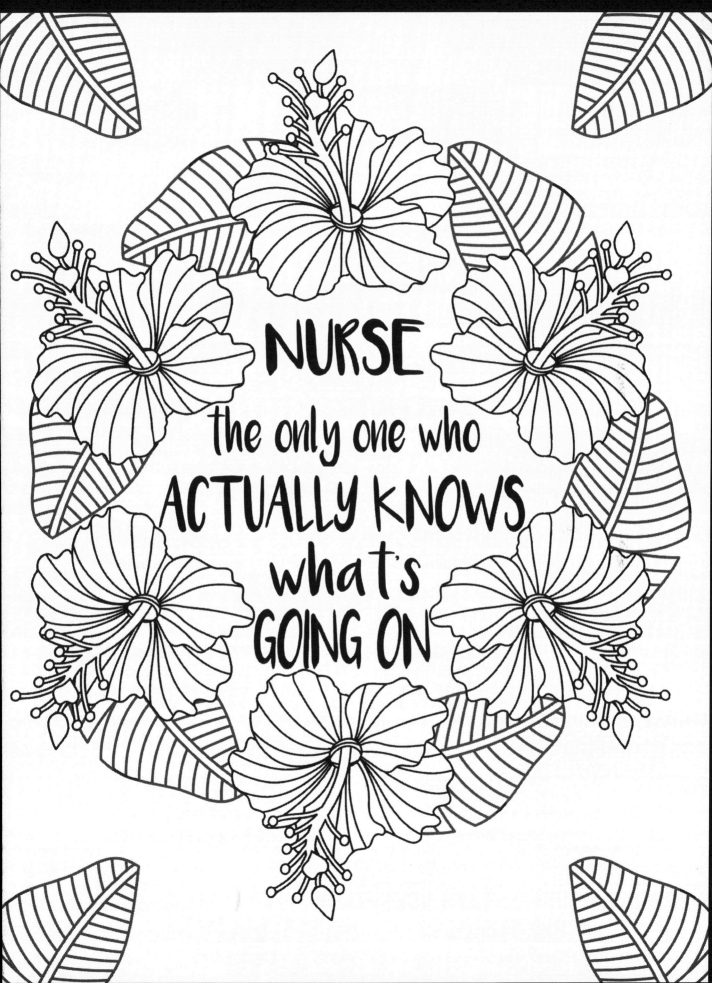

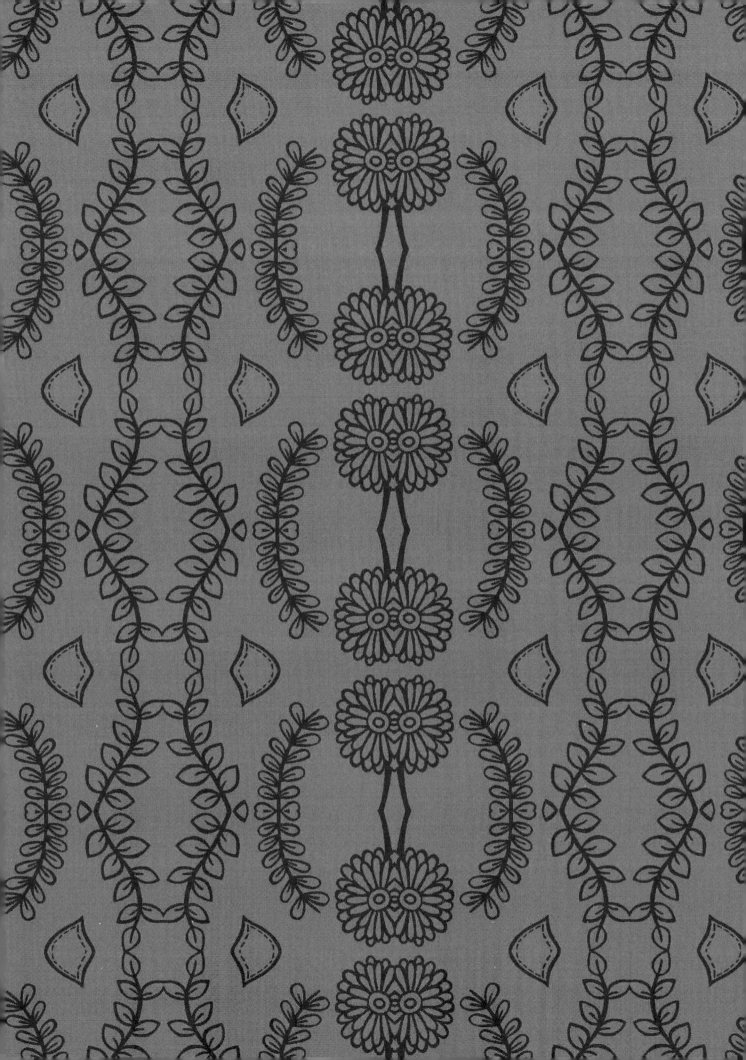

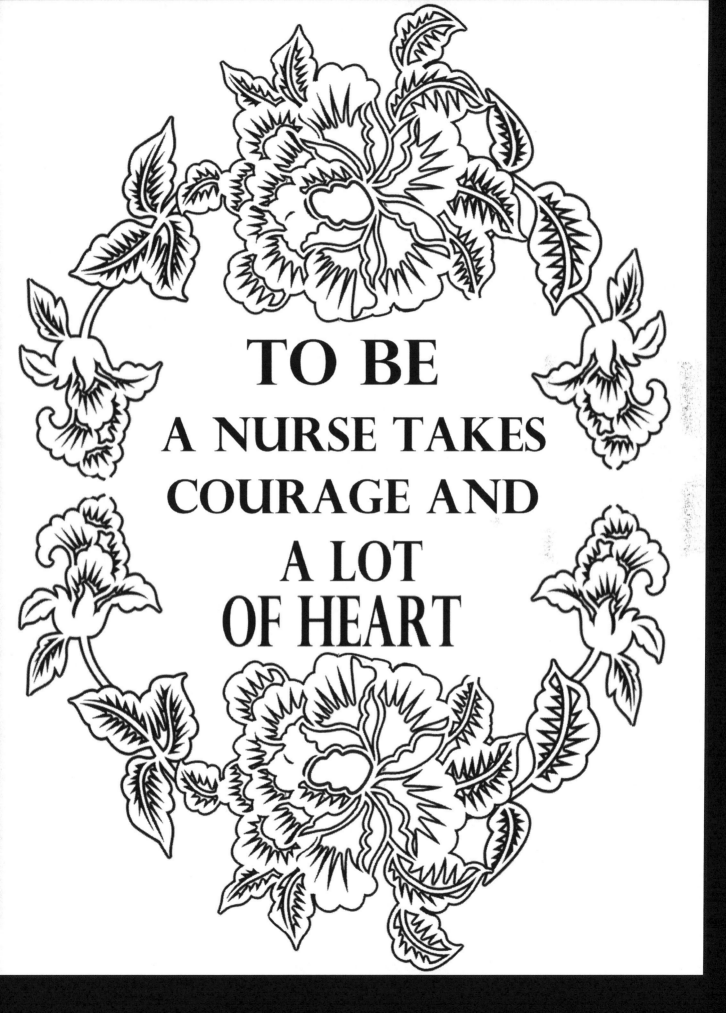

TO BE
A NURSE TAKES
COURAGE AND
A LOT
OF HEART

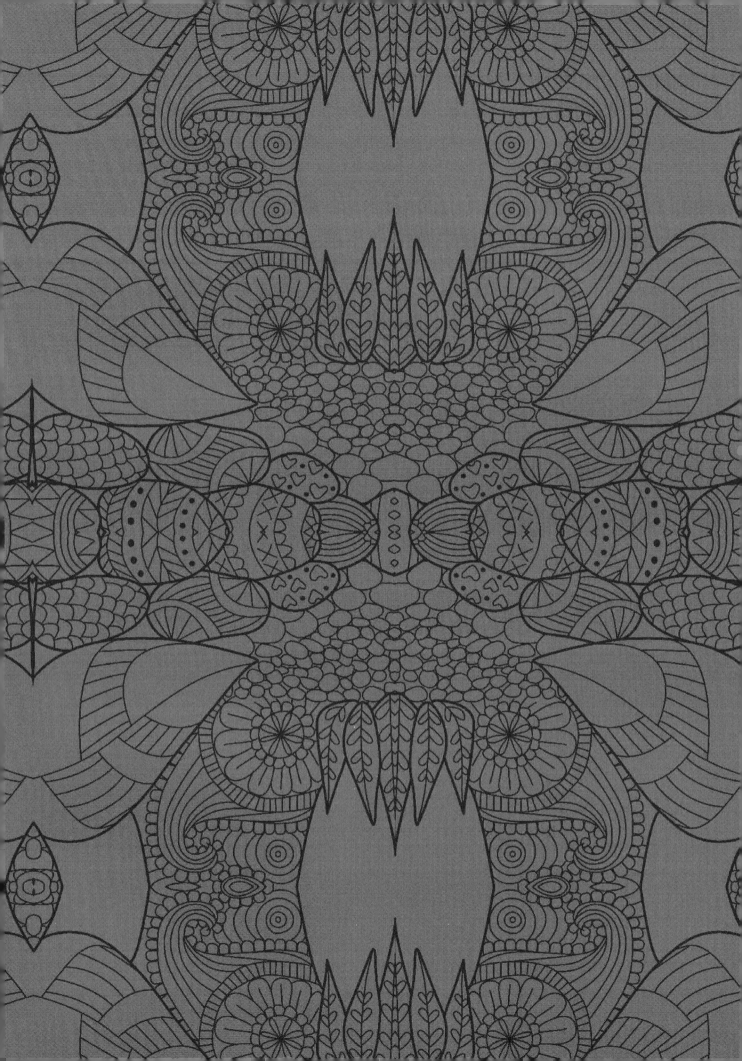

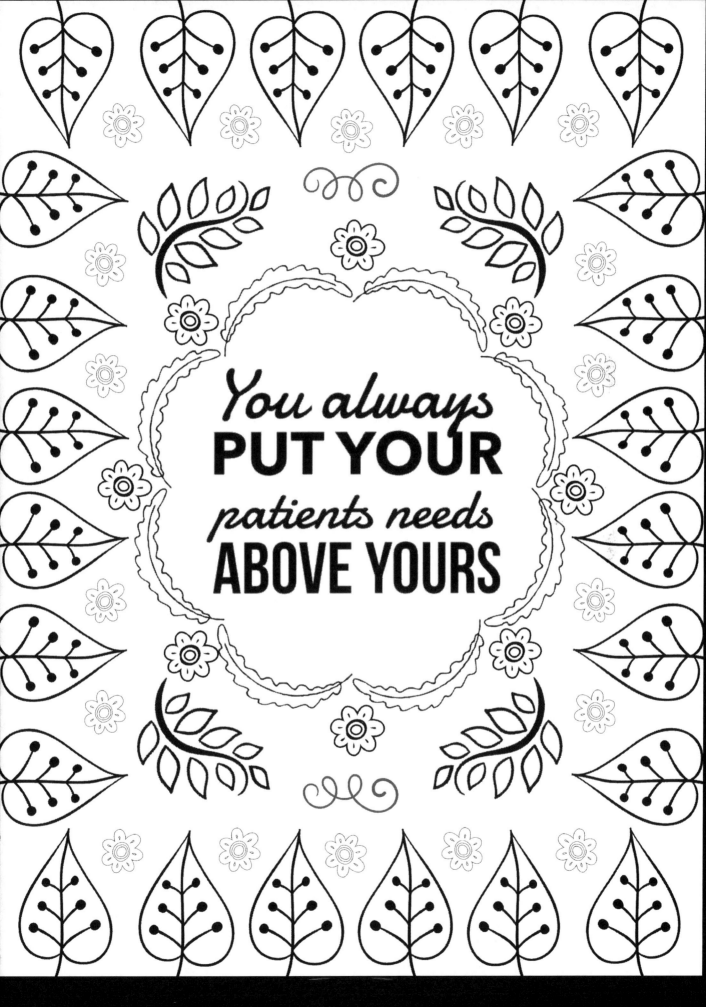

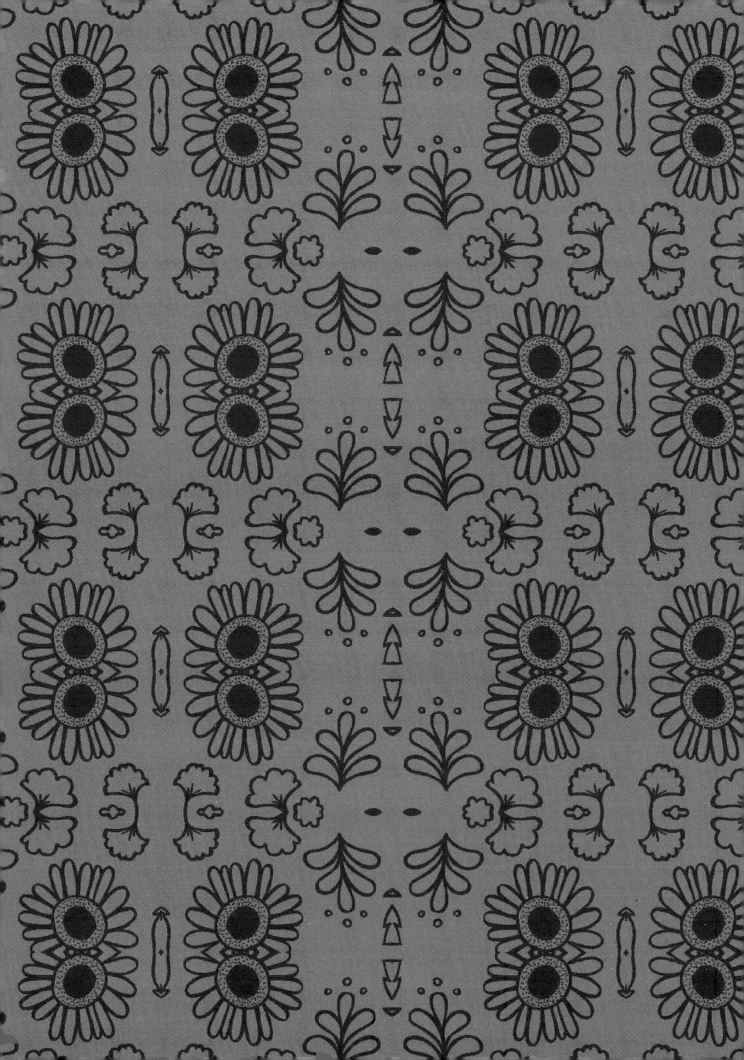

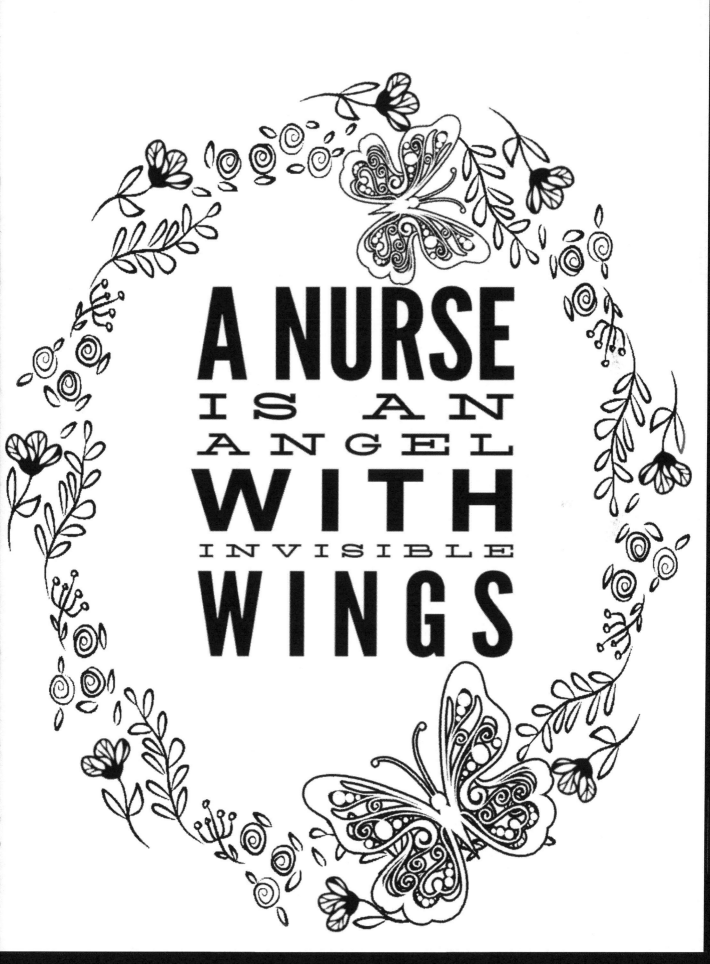

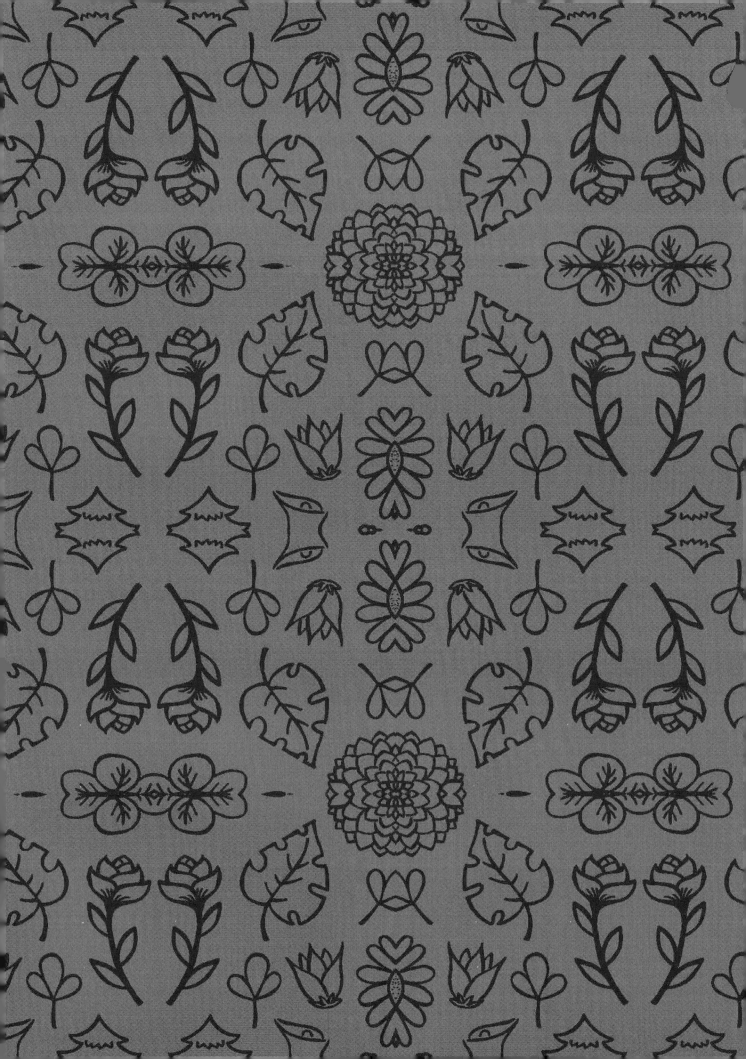

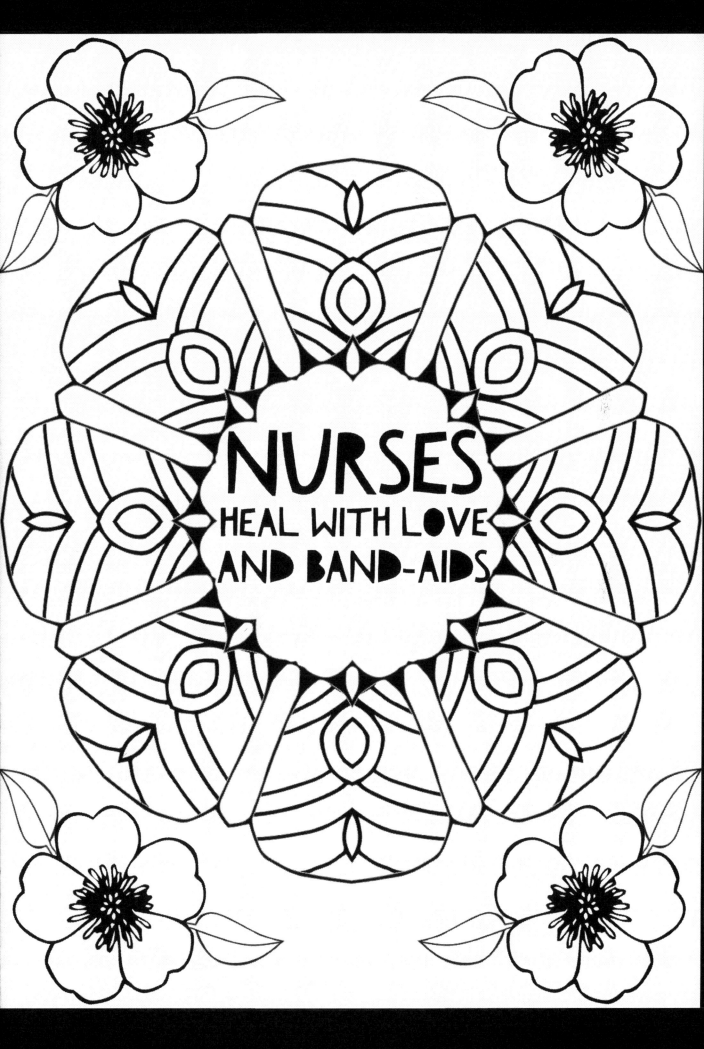

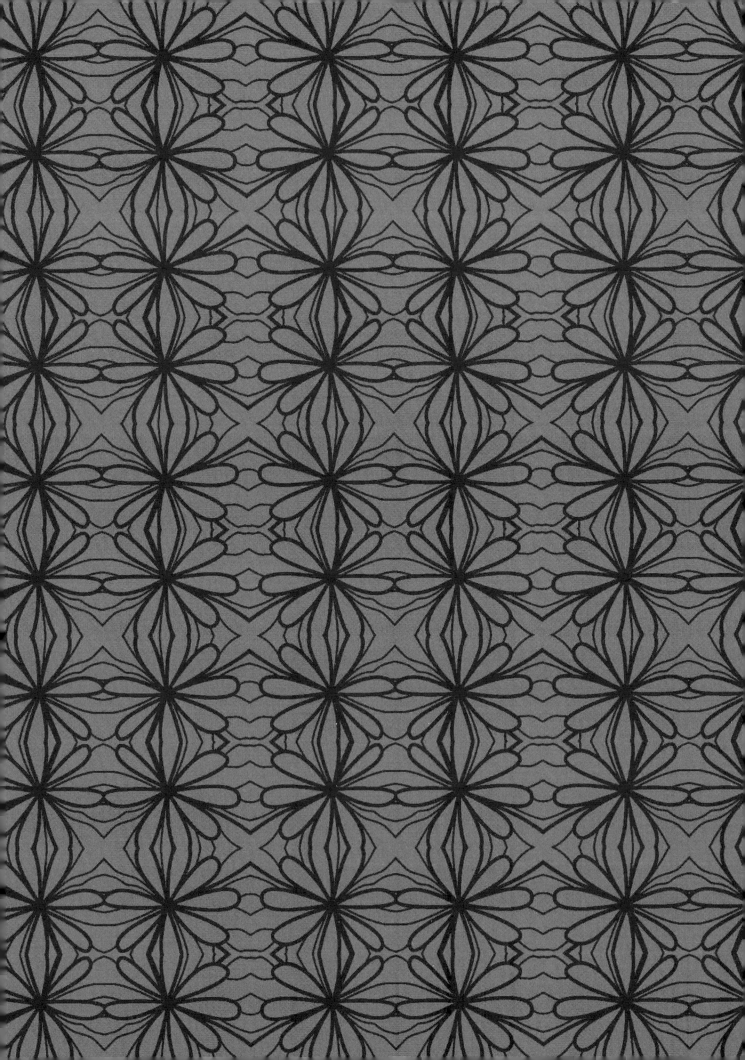

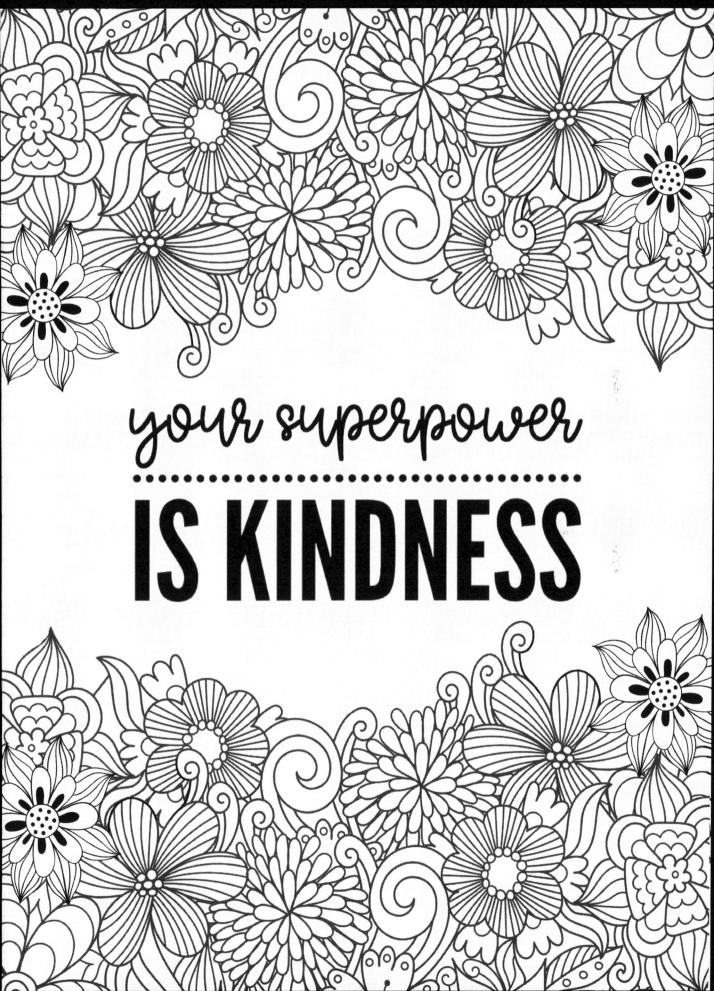

your superpower
··
IS KINDNESS

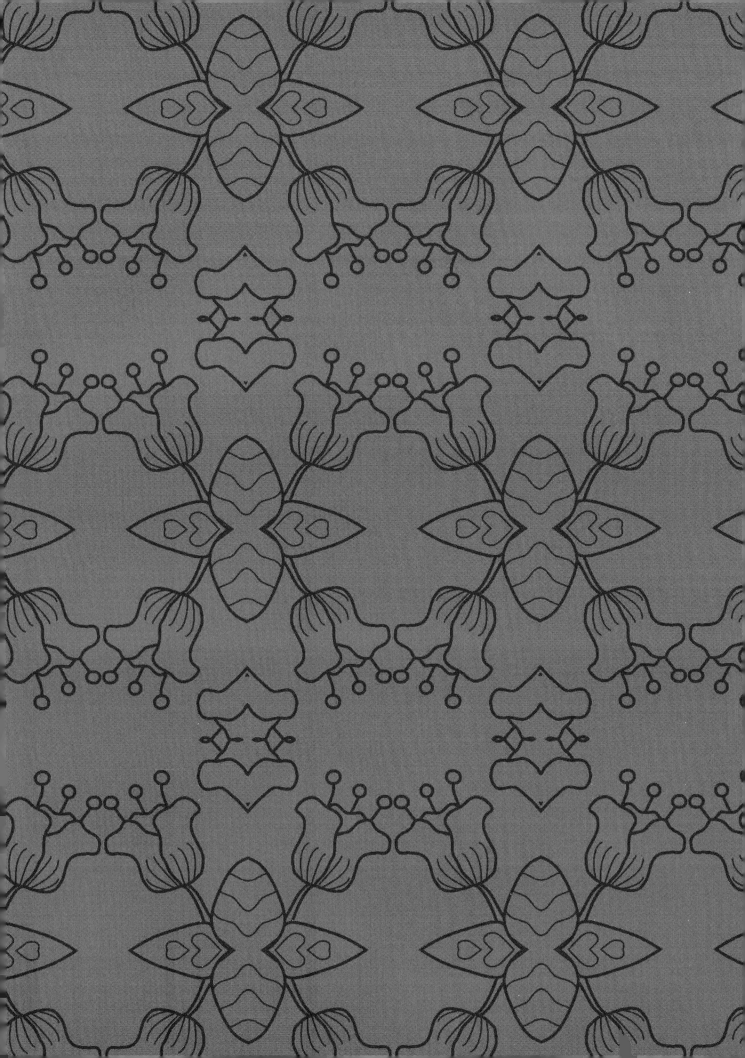

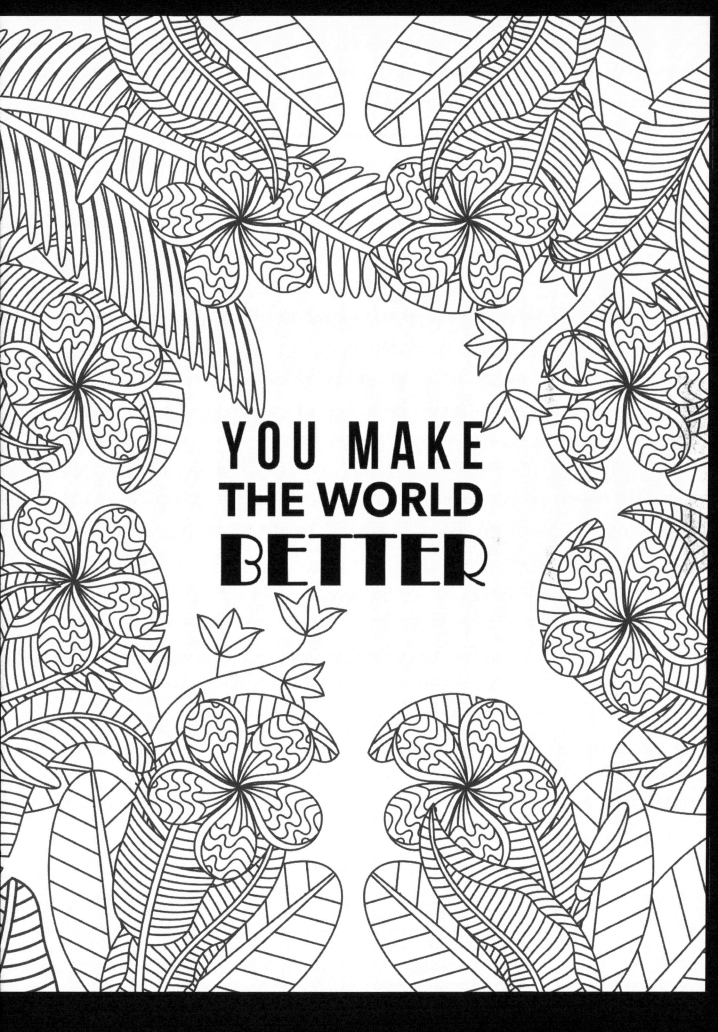

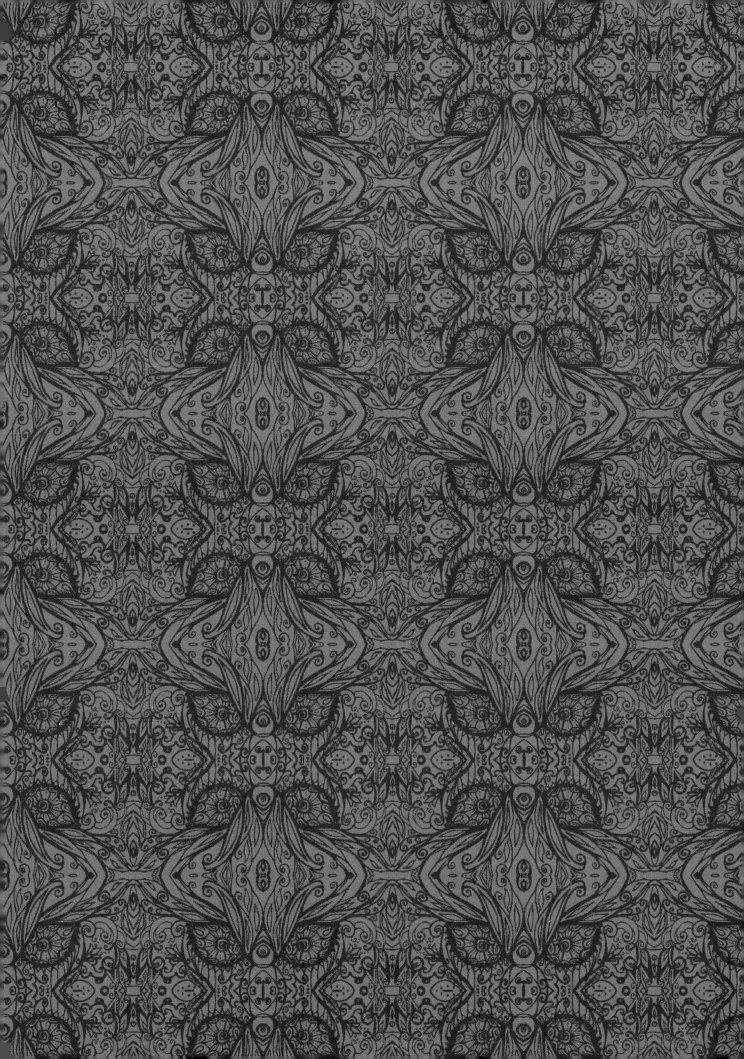

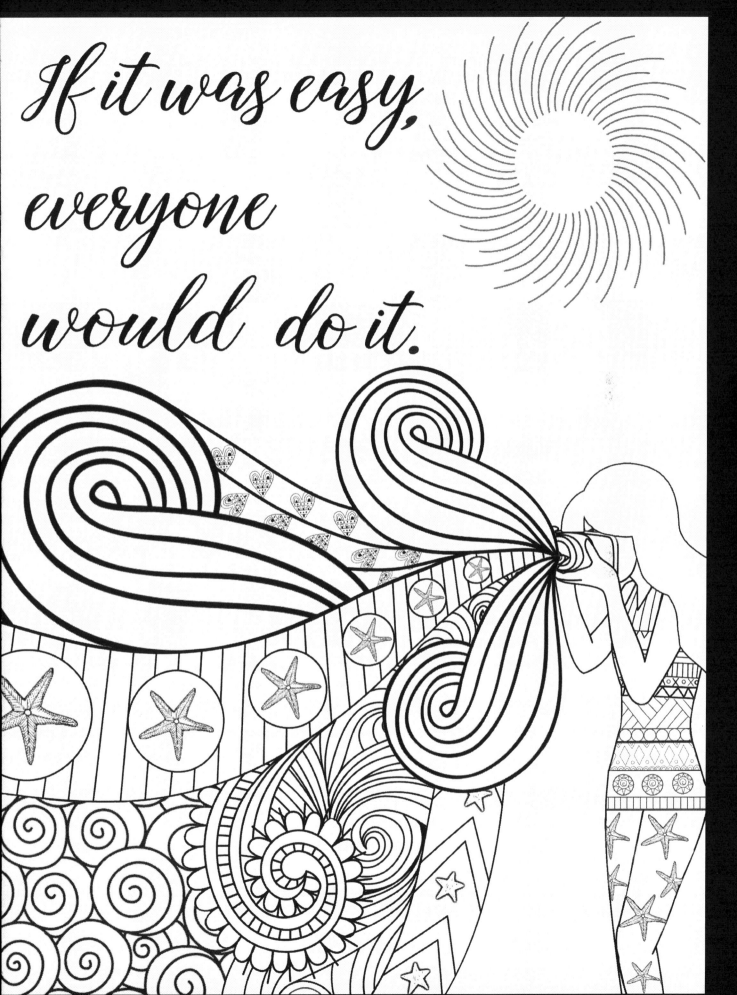

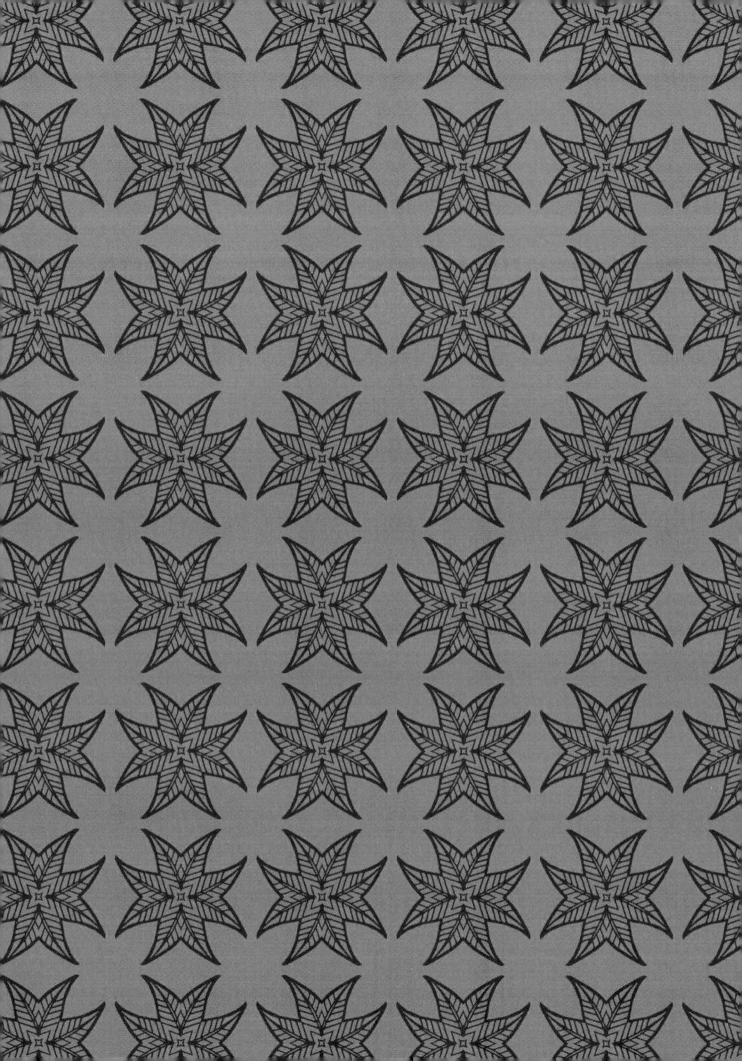

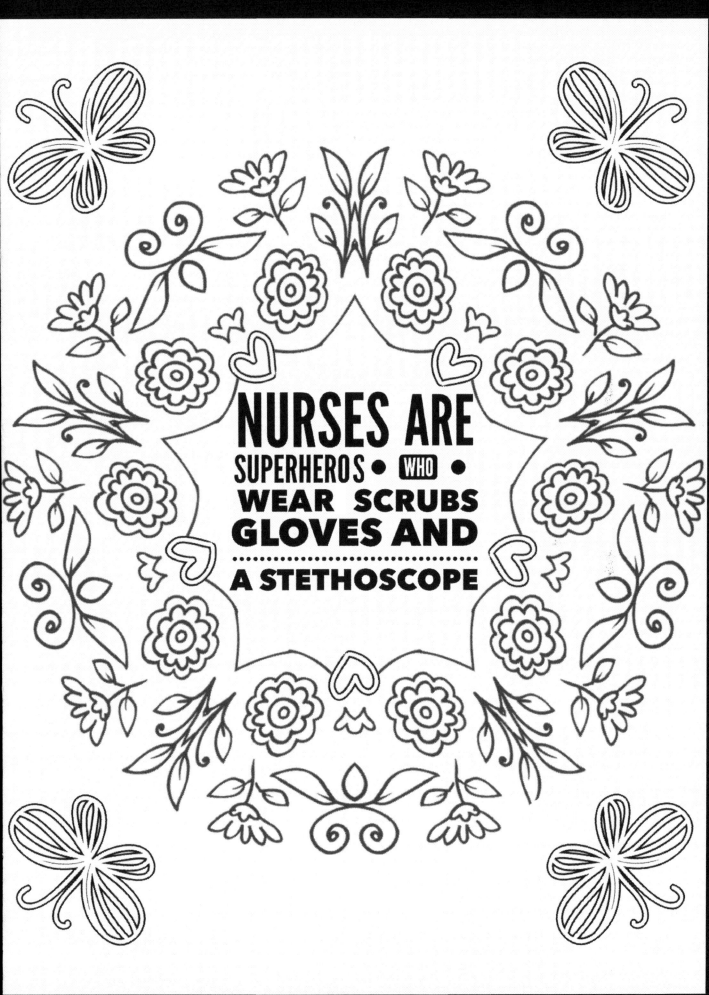

NURSES ARE SUPERHEROS • WHO • WEAR SCRUBS GLOVES AND A STETHOSCOPE

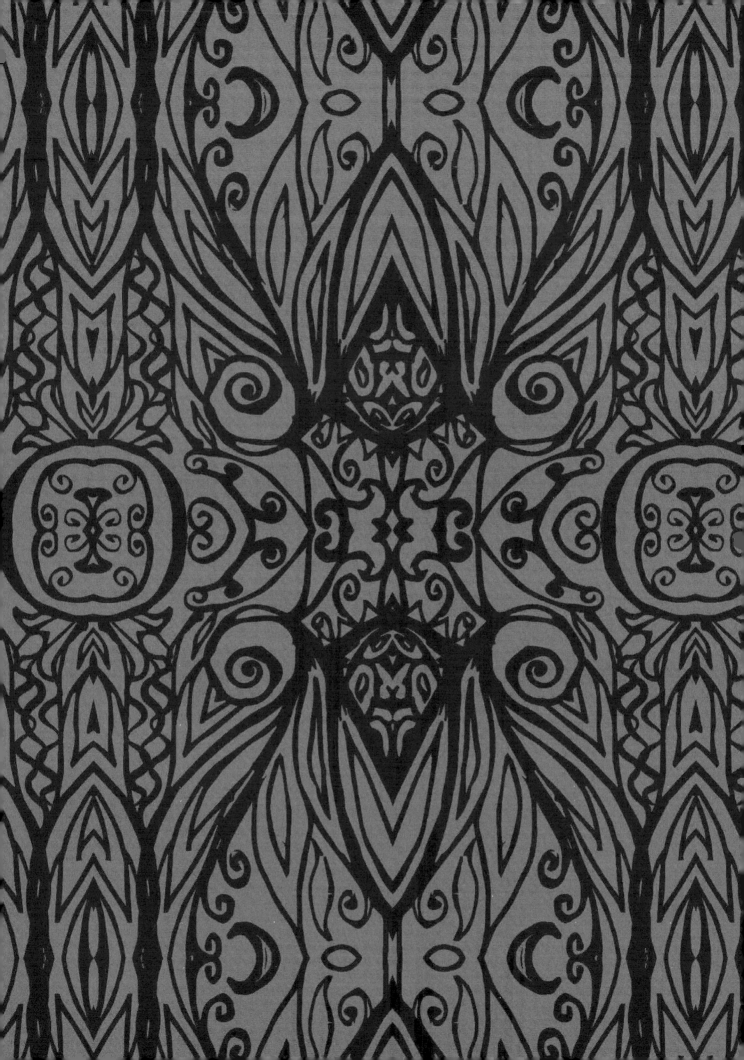

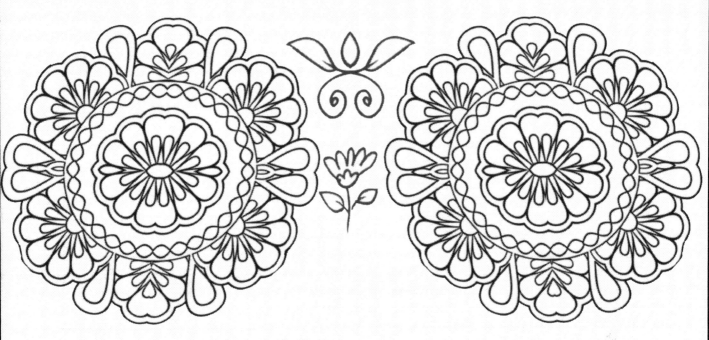

KEEP CALM
AND THINK LIKE

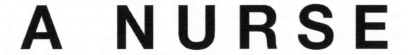

A NURSE

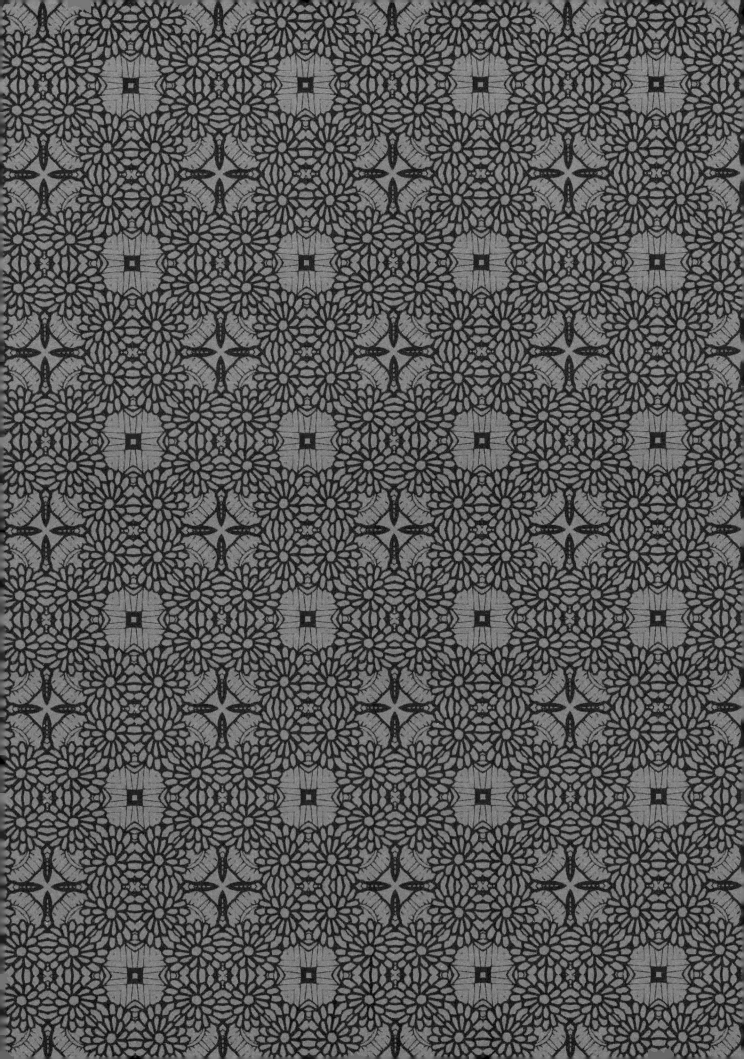

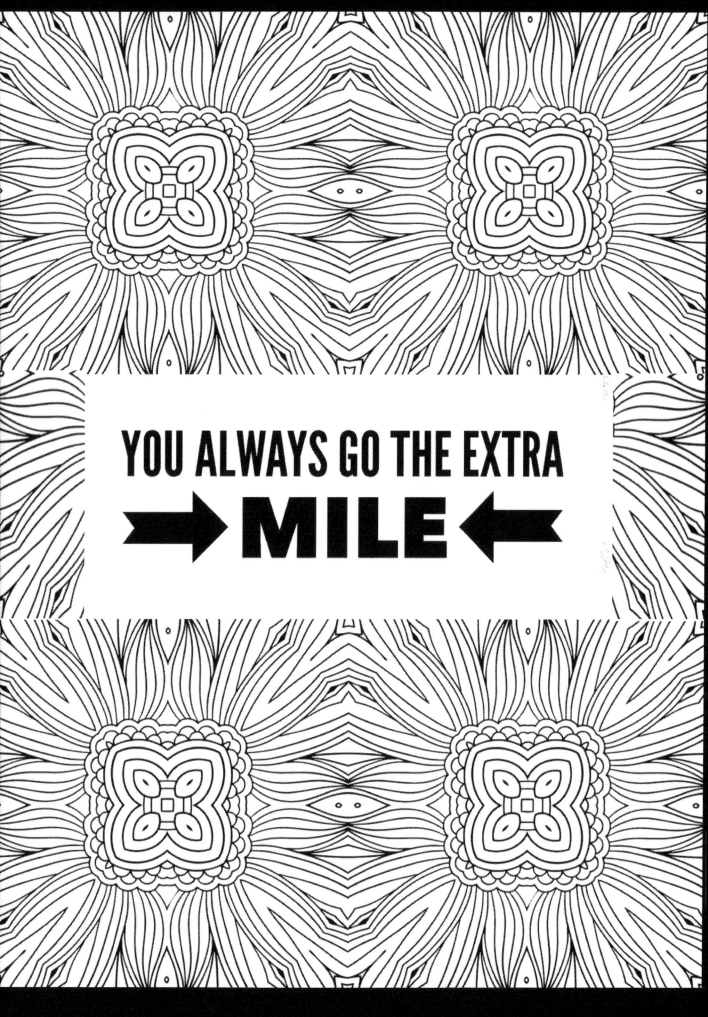

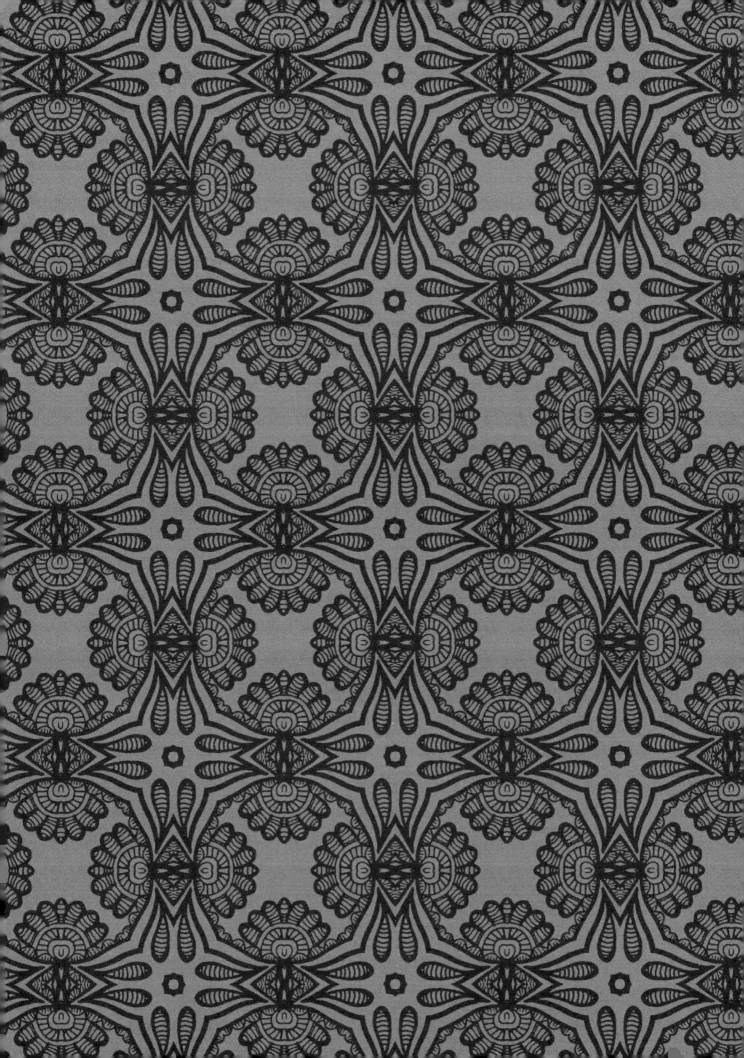

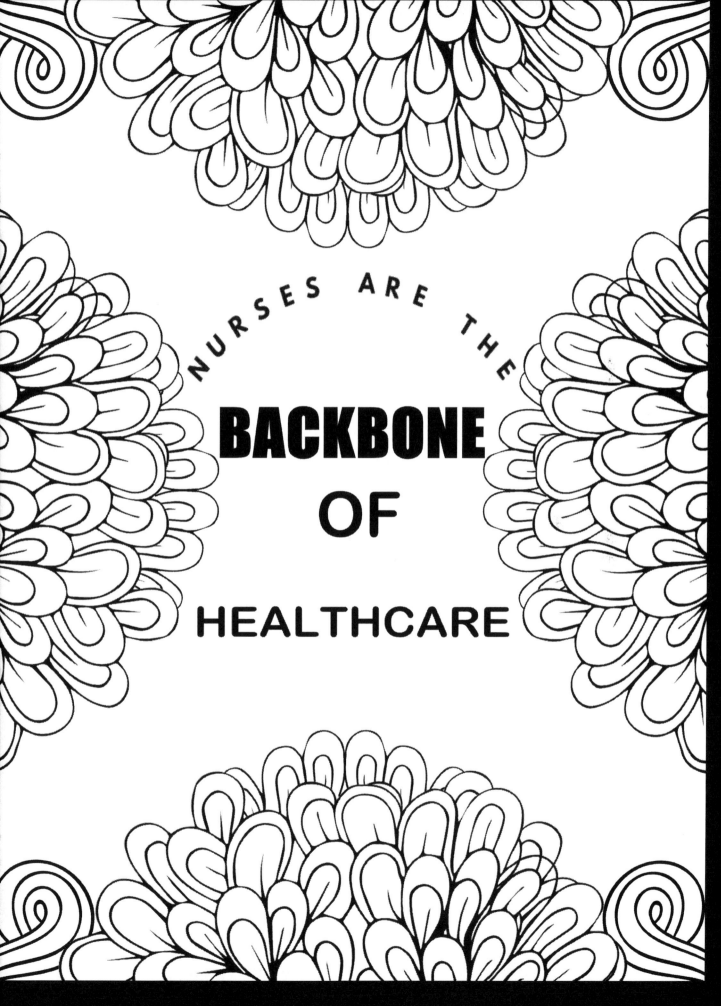

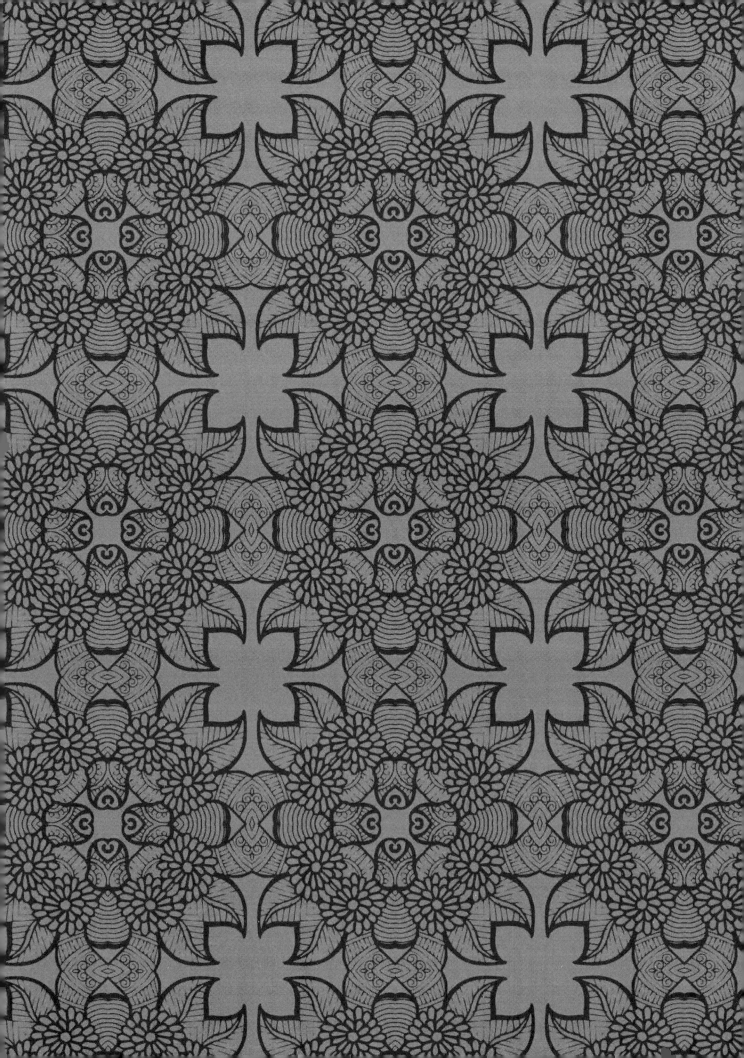

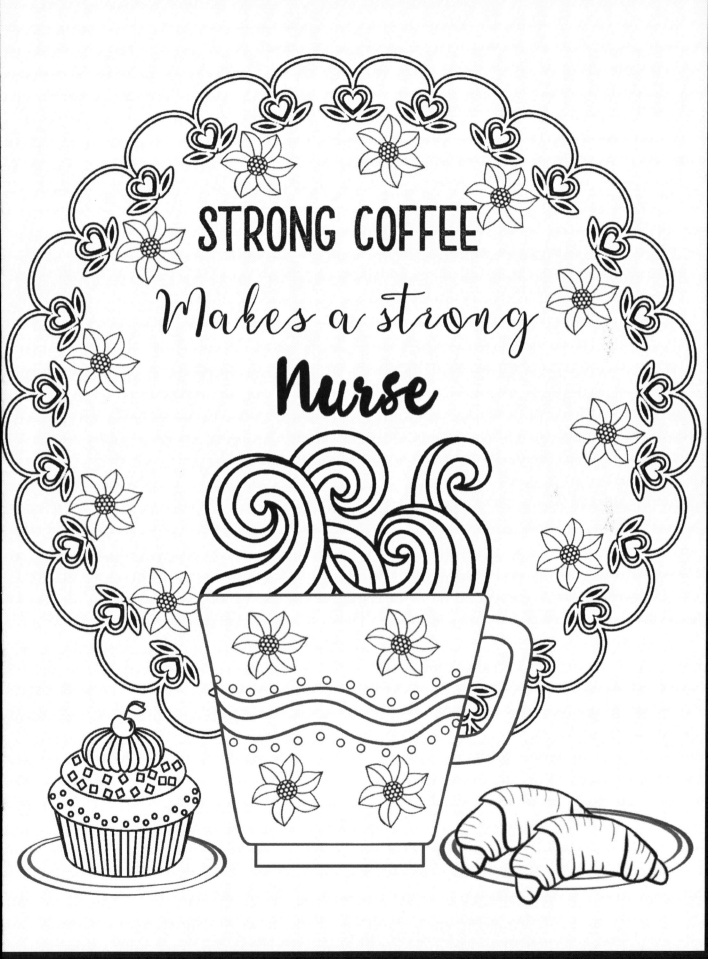

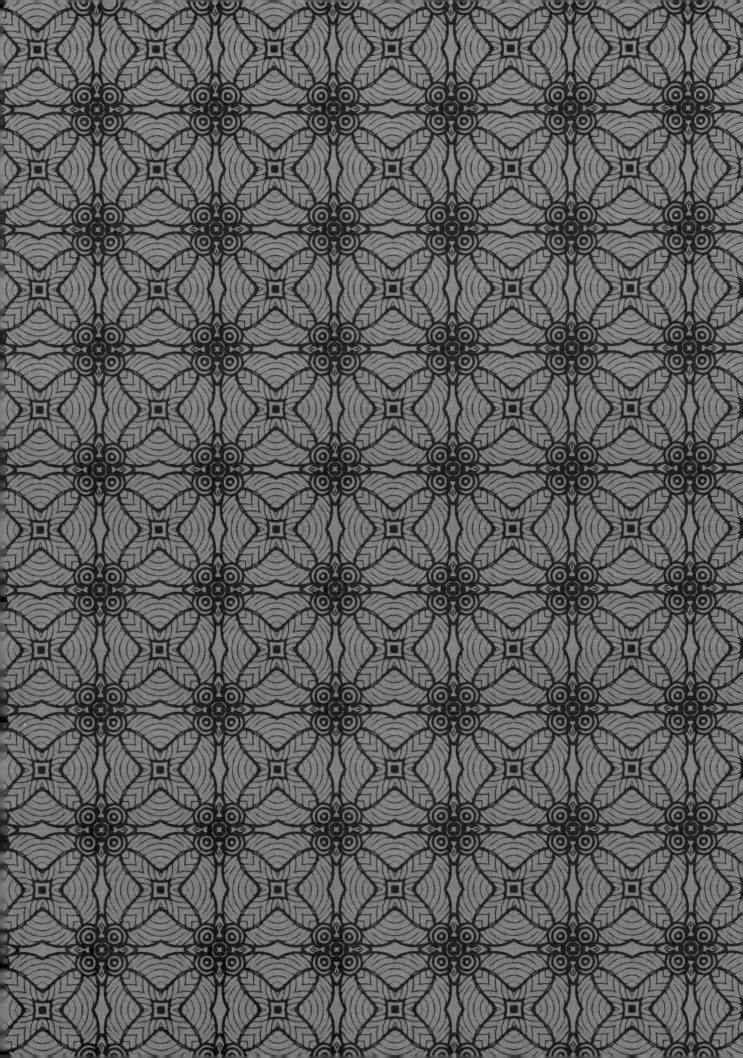

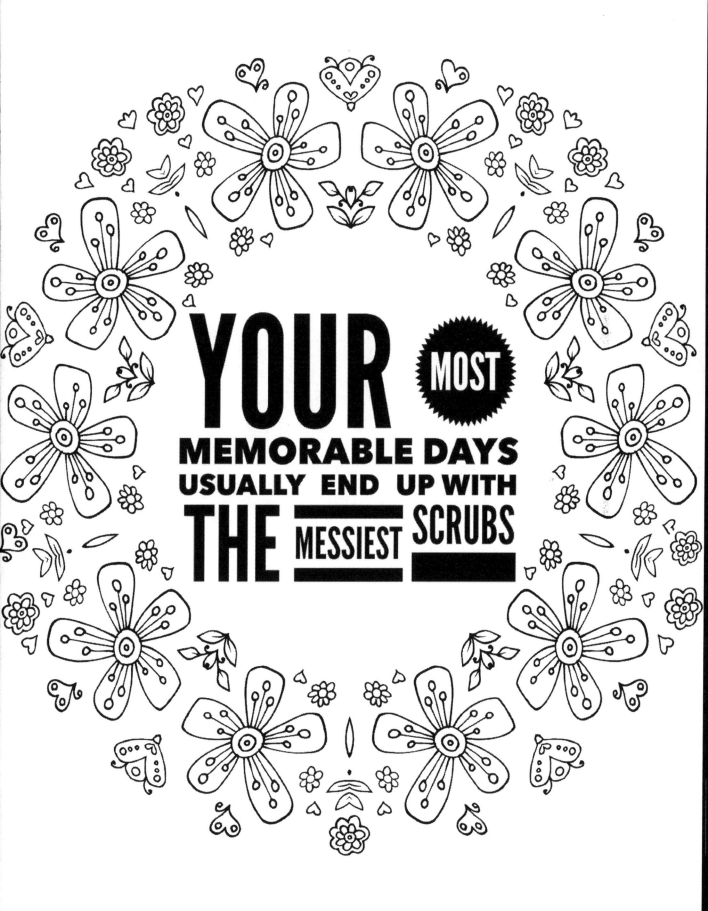

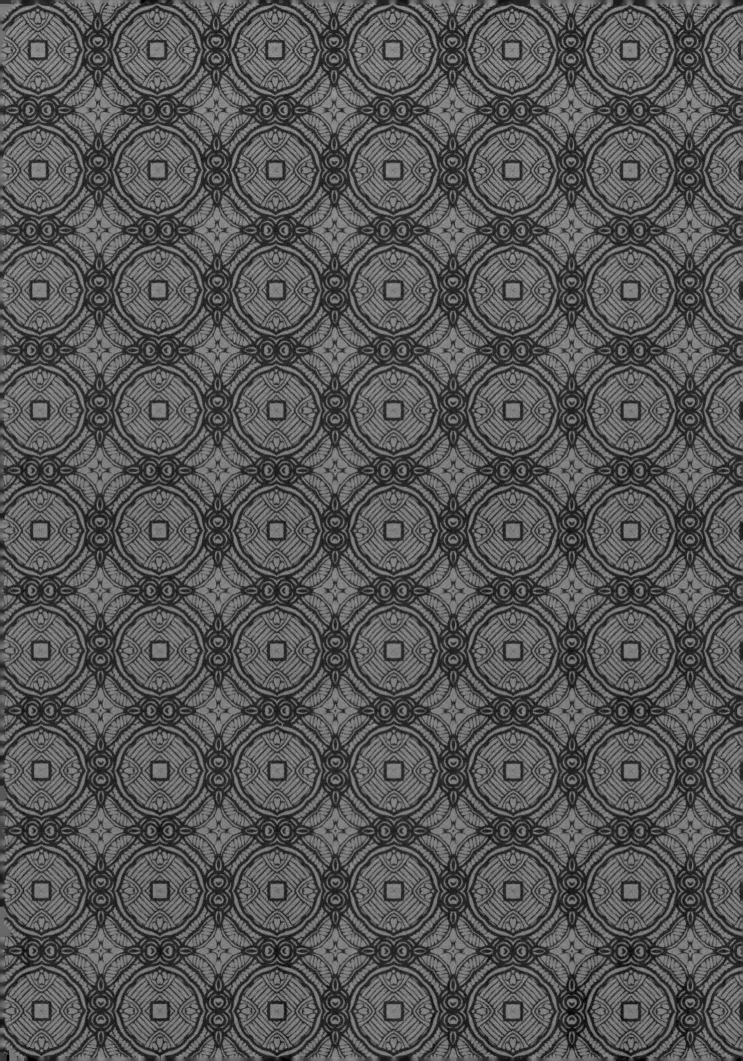

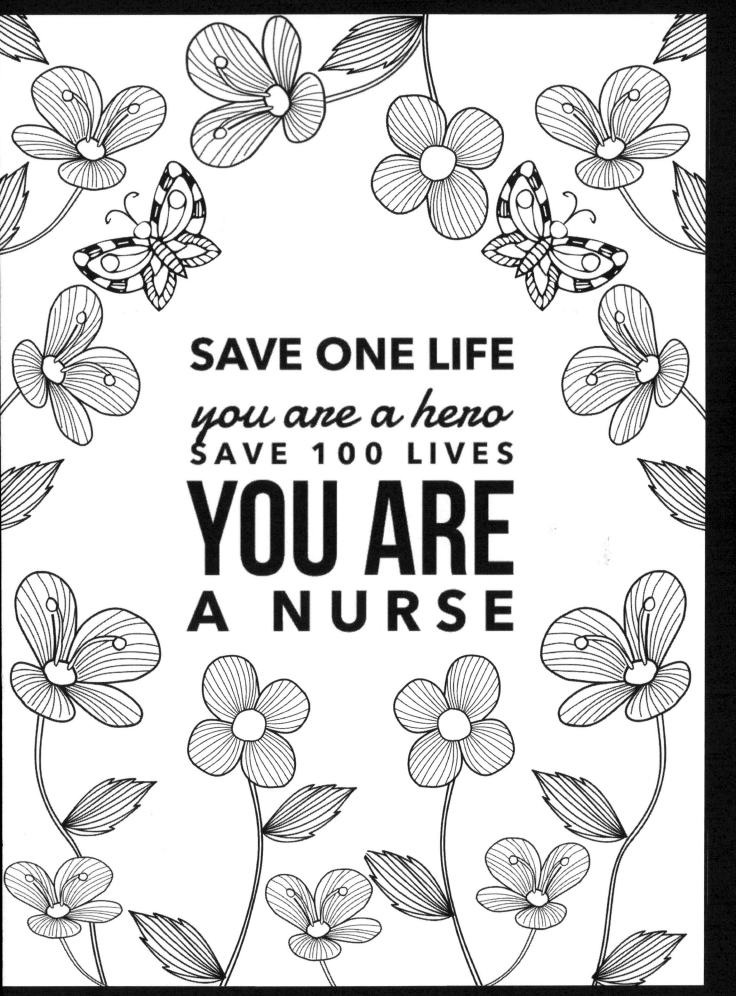

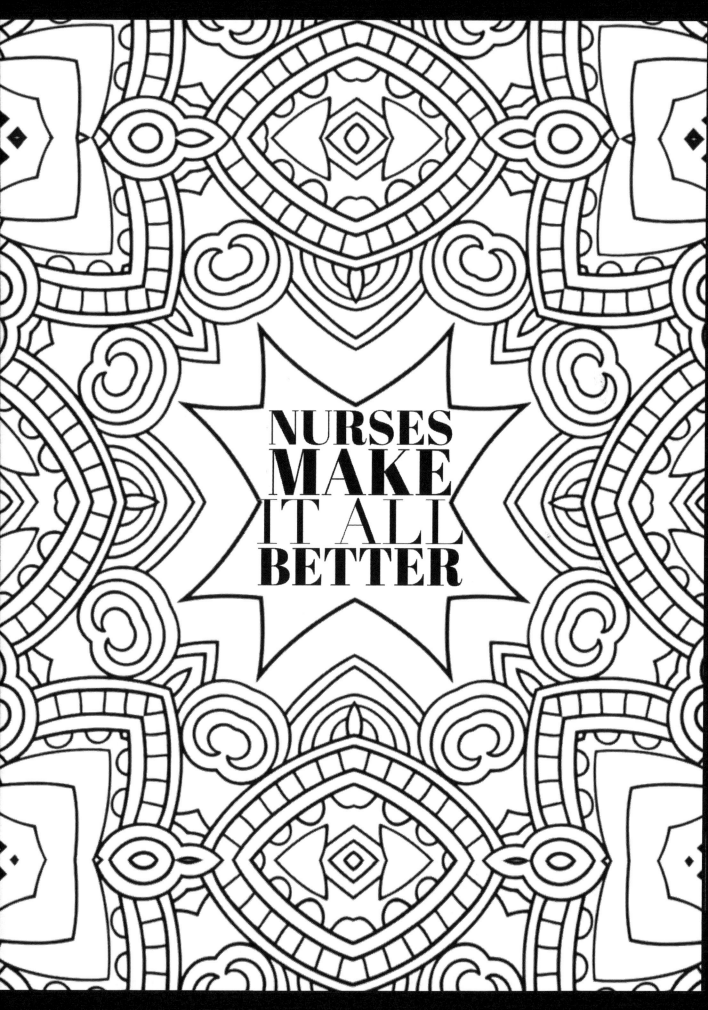

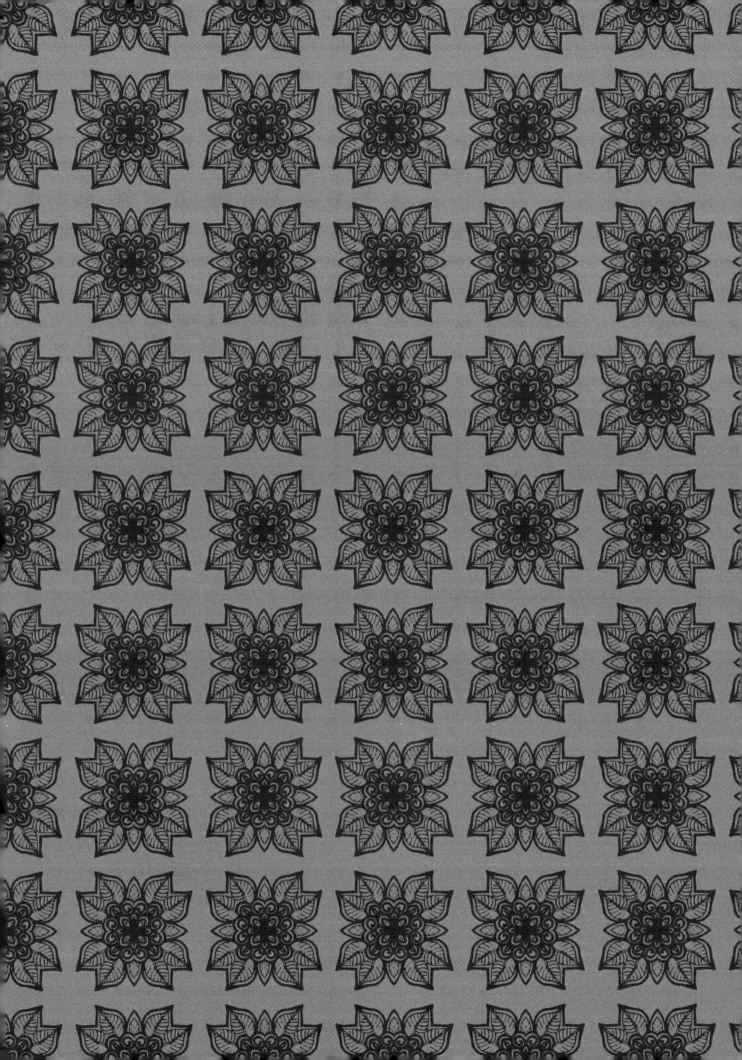

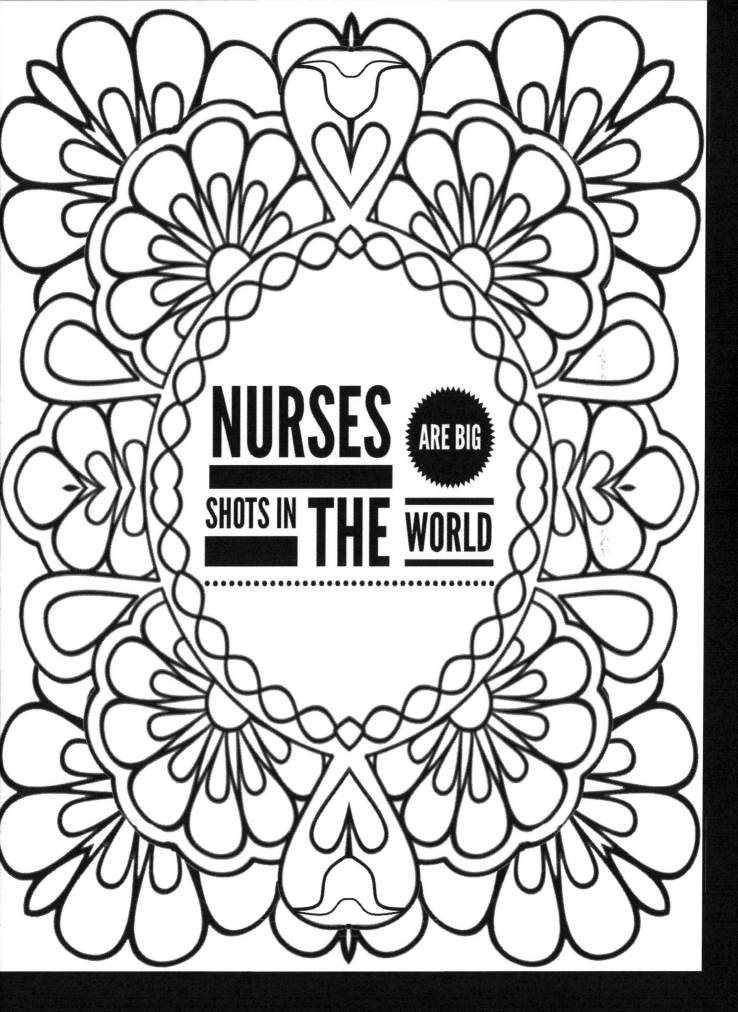

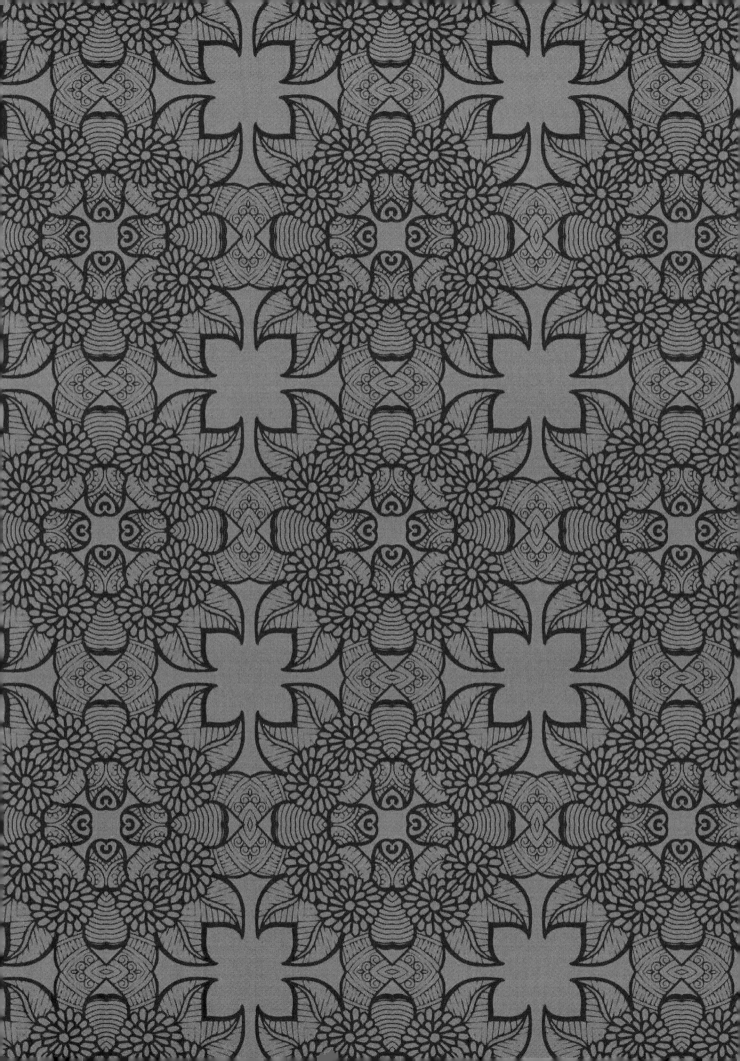

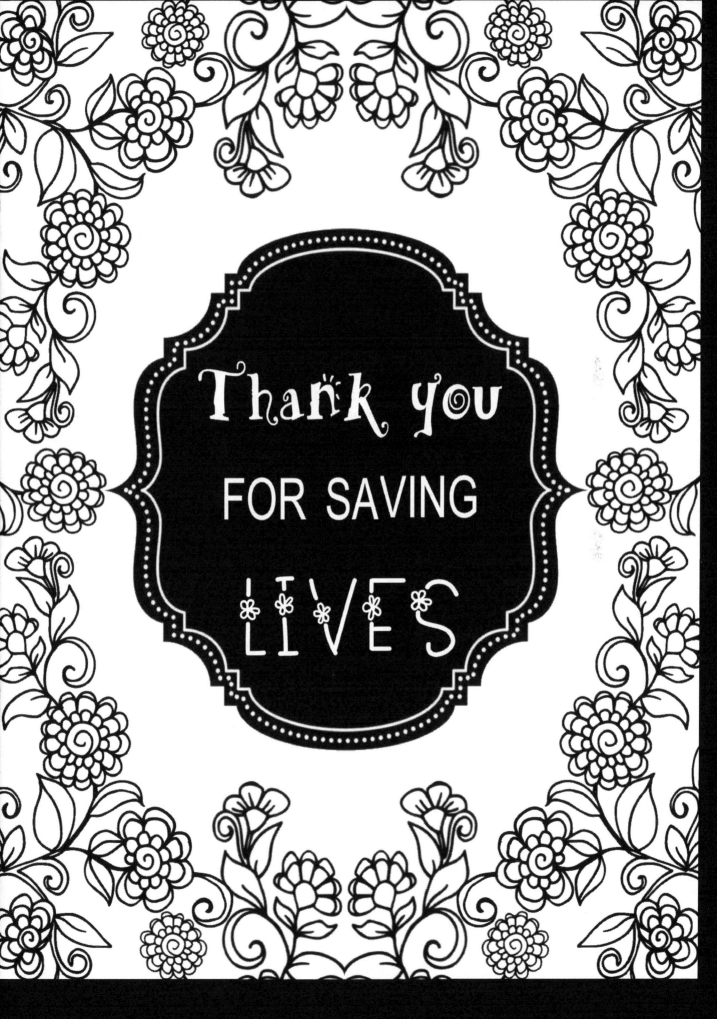

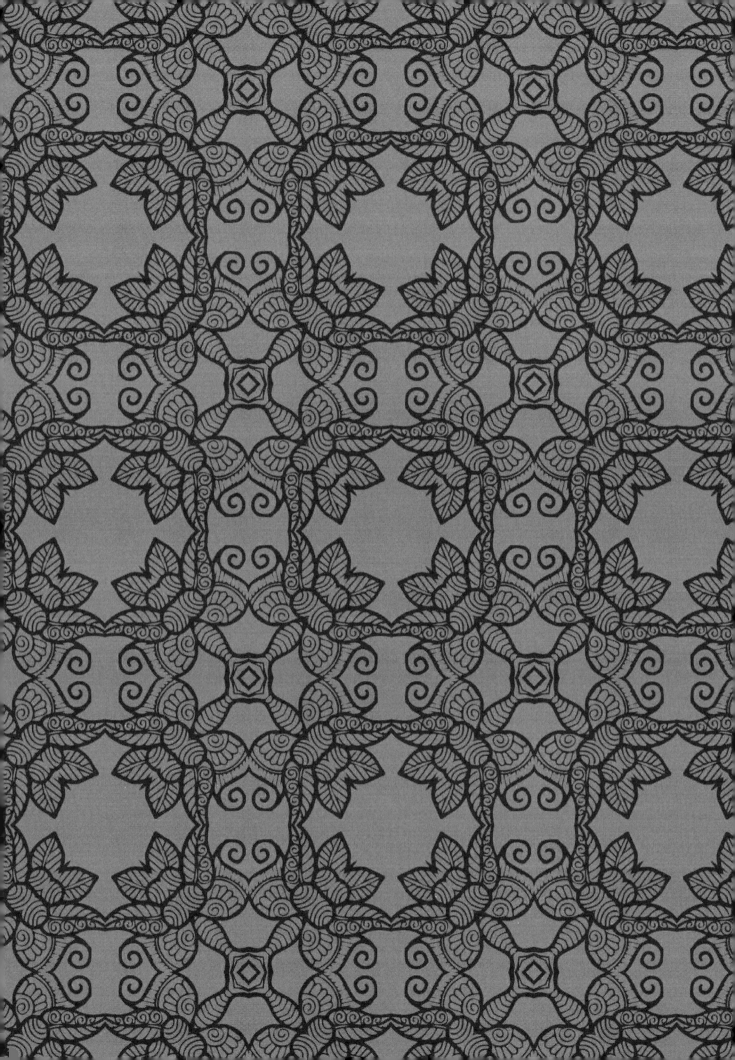

Hello,

We would like to take a moment and thank all the wonderful nurses for their devotion and hard work to take care of each and every patient.

We hope you enjoy this book and would love your feed back.

Please write us a review for "Nurse coloring book" author by Noah's Art at Amazon.com

Thank you,

Noah's Art Team.

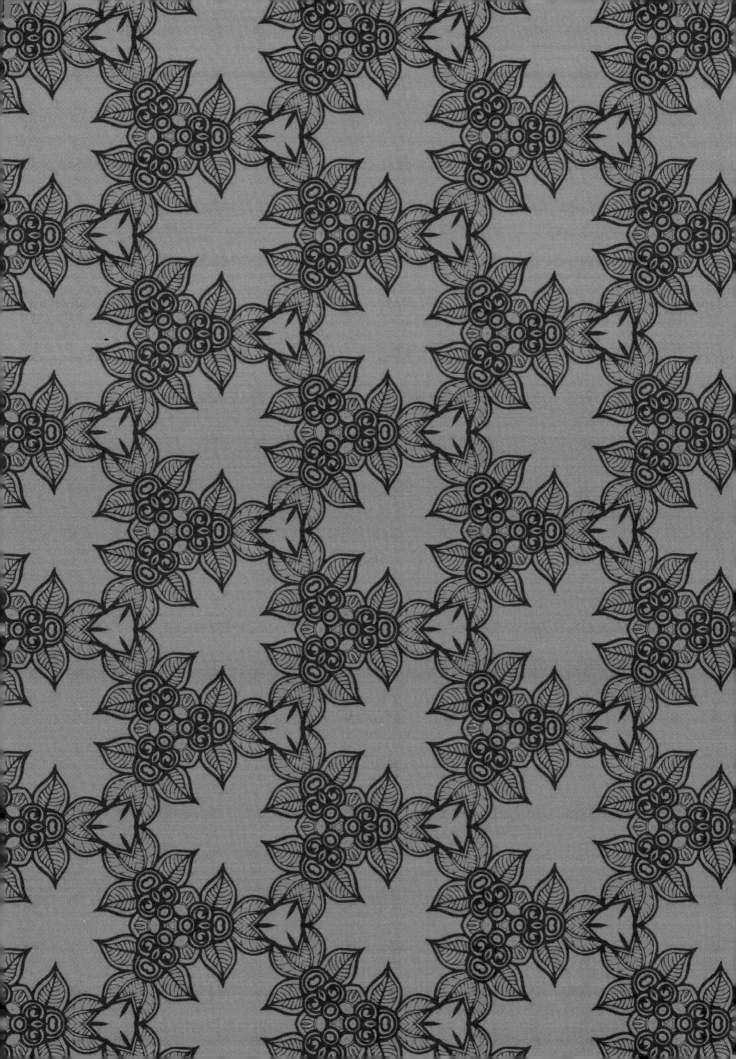

COLOR TEST PAGE

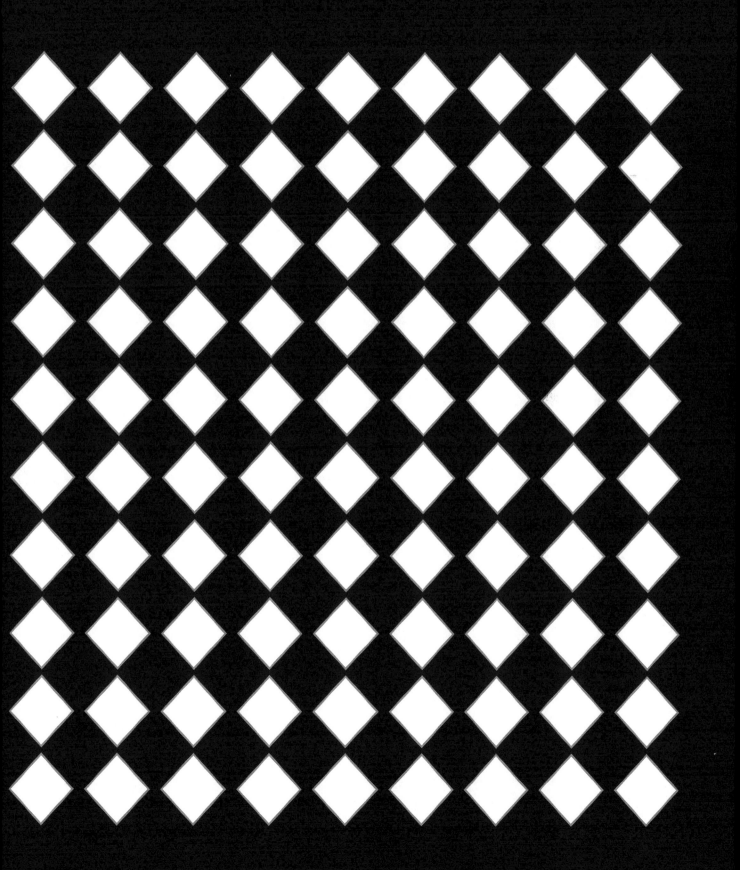

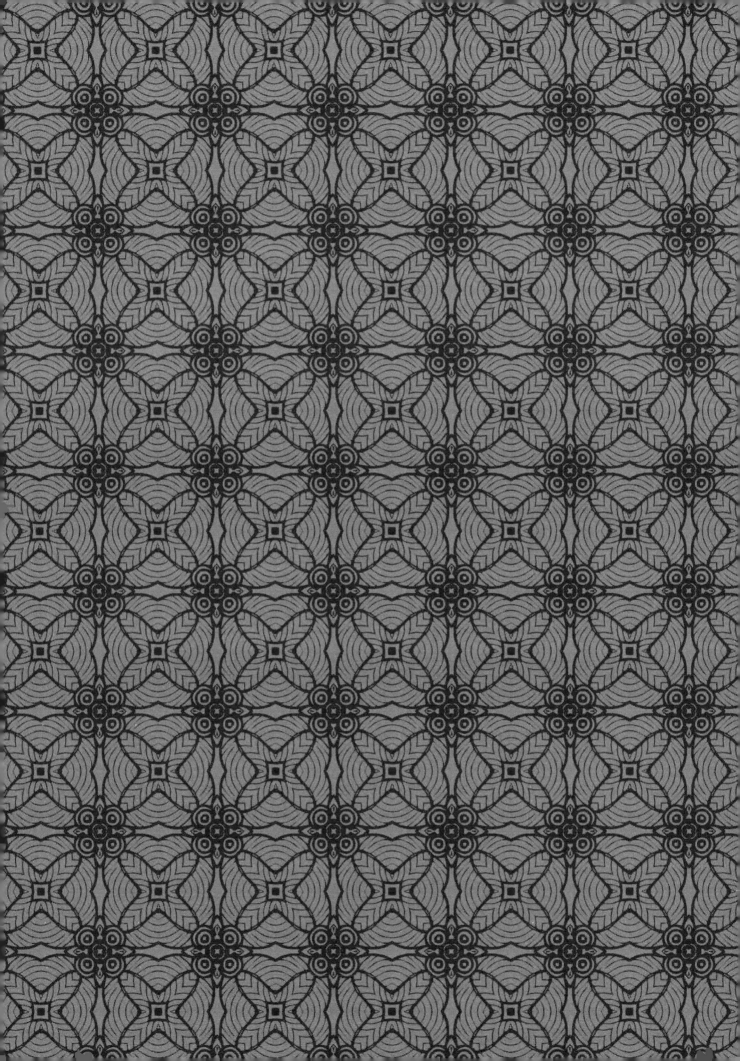

COLOR TEST PAGE

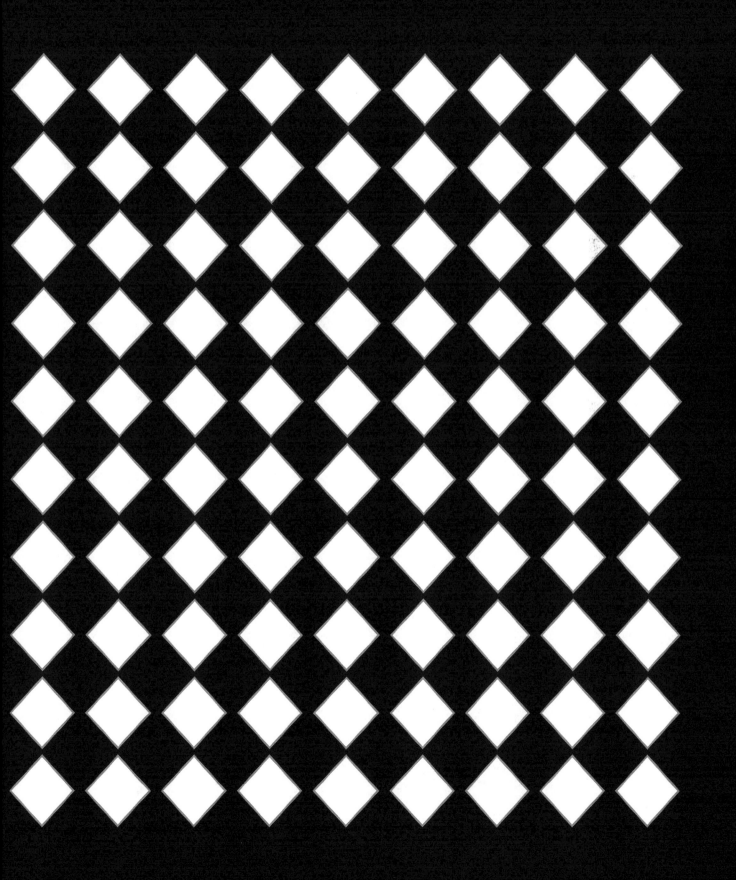

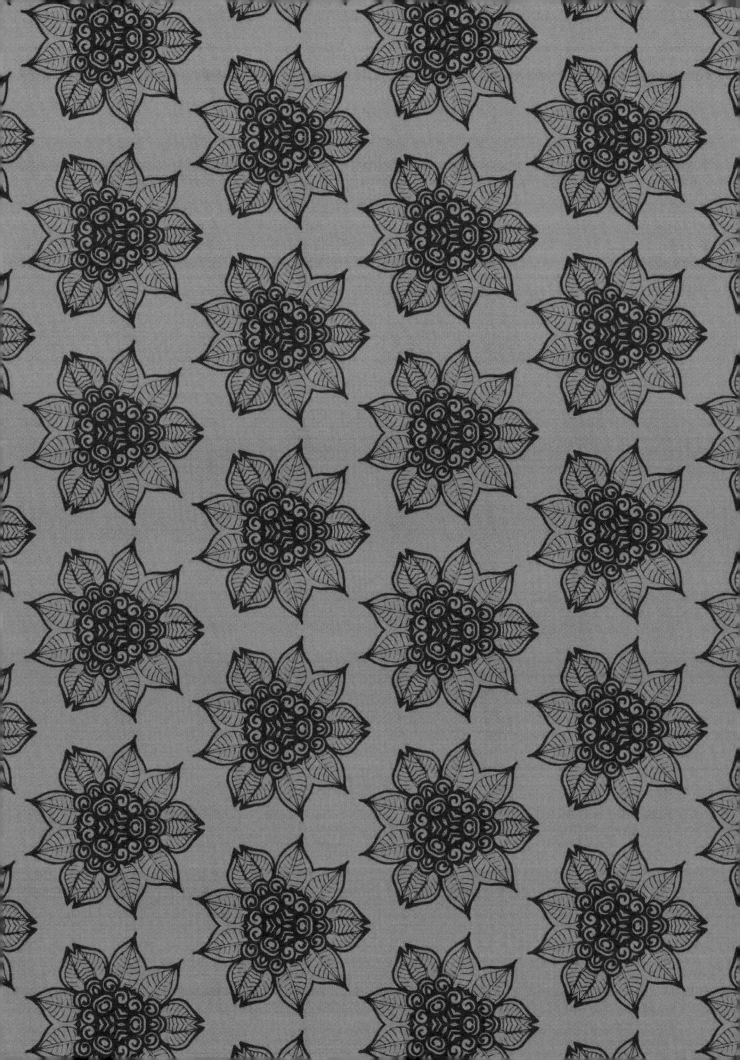

Made in the USA
San Bernardino, CA
16 December 2019